Lunatics, Imbeciles and Idiots

Lunatics, Imbeciles and Idiots

A History of Insanity in Nineteenth-Century Britain and Ireland

Kathryn M. Burtinshaw
and John R.F. Burt

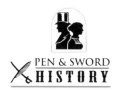

PEN & SWORD
HISTORY

First published in Great Britain in 2017 by
PEN AND SWORD HISTORY
an imprint of
Pen and Sword Books Ltd
47 Church Street
Barnsley
South Yorkshire S70 2AS

ISBN 978 1 47387 903 4

A CIP record for this book is available from the British Library

Printed and bound in England
by CPI Group (UK) Ltd, Croydon, CR0 4YY

Typeset in Times New Roman by Chic Graphics

Pen & Sword Books Ltd incorporates the imprints of Pen & Sword
Archaeology, Atlas, Aviation, Battleground, Discovery,
Family History, History, Maritime, Military, Naval, Politics, Railways,
Select, Social History, Transport, True Crime, Claymore Press,
Frontline Books, Leo Cooper, Praetorian Press, Remember When,
Seaforth Publishing and Wharncliffe.

For a complete list of Pen and Sword titles please contact
Pen and Sword Books Limited
47 Church Street, Barnsley, South Yorkshire, S70 2AS, England
E-mail: enquiries@pen-and-sword.co.uk
Website: www.pen-and-sword.co.uk

Contents

Acknowledgements

We would like to extend our grateful thanks to Caroline Brown, Programme Leader and University Archivist at The Centre for Archive and Information Studies (CAIS), University of Dundee – she inspired us from the start and has been invaluable in assisting us with providing information and imagery. Thanks also to Dr Louise Williams, Archivist at Lothian Health Services Archive and the staff at The Centre for Research Collections at the University of Edinburgh Library.

Appreciation is extended to the staff at Cheshire Archives in Chester; Denbighshire Archives at Ruthin; The National Records of Scotland; and The National Library of Scotland in Edinburgh; Archives and Special Collections at University of Stirling Library; The Heritage Hub in Hawick; and The Public Record Office of Northern Ireland (PRONI) in Belfast.

We thank Aedan Burt and Susannah Burtinshaw for their willingness to proofread this book.

We are most grateful to Karyn Burnham who made a number of invaluable, helpful and constructive comments in editing an earlier version of this book.

Introduction

The title of this book *Lunatics, Imbeciles and Idiots* is provocative – yet these terms were regularly used to label people with mental health disorders in nineteenth century Britain and Ireland. These archaic and confrontational definitions, which in today's society are totally unacceptable, had concise medical definitions in the nineteenth century and were in common usage in their day.

At the start of the nineteenth century there was neglect of, and surprisingly little control over, the provision of care for individuals suffering from mental health problems. Prior to this, individuals who were considered insane or mentally deficient were often treated in an appalling way with little or no thought to their likely recovery. They were chained up in outhouses, or cells in gaols, prisons or workhouses and treated as wild animals. People suffering from congenital disorders such as Down's syndrome or cretinism, deaf mutes and epileptics were all included in this incarceration.

At the beginning of the nineteenth century a group of philanthropic and influential people recognised the genuine predicament of those considered to be insane. An understanding developed that these people were human beings who, through little fault of their own, had become the most vulnerable class of society in Great Britain and Ireland. The derangement of their mind, either from birth or acquired through injury or illness, was a condition that should be cared for and where possible treated. With this realisation, the authorities gradually brought about change. Their new belief was that asylums were required as 'institutions for the shelter and support of afflicted or destitute persons, in particular … the insane'. Gradually this led to the proper establishment of a network of pauper asylums throughout the United Kingdom. Dr W.A.F. Browne, Superintendent of the Montrose Royal Lunatic Asylum, set out a framework and missionary statement in his seminal work *What Asylums Were, Are, and Ought to Be* in 1837.

New legislation significantly altered the manner in which those with mental health disorders were treated. Manacles and chains were discarded and a caring approach to treatment was adopted. Squalid, dirty and prison like conditions were abandoned and curative accommodation in hospital-like surroundings was provided. It was recognised that some mental health disorders could be alleviated by a humane approach to their care and those with problems began to be treated less like animals and more like real people who had rights, hopes and a desire to be well.

In many respects improved legislation also altered public perception about people who had previously been deemed 'abnormal'. The new asylums of the nineteenth century were considered to be curative shelters for people that society did not understand, but they also became places where a new class of health professional, the 'mad doctor', 'alienist' or as we term it today 'psychiatrist' was trying to understand human mental affliction and finding ways to alleviate or cure it.

However, as new public asylums increased in number and size, so did the number of patients requiring their assistance. Debilitated by a variety of mental and behavioural difficulties such as epilepsy, melancholia, mania, general paralysis or dementia, these people were admitted to asylums in the hope of care, cure and comfort.

The nineteenth century is recognised as a century of record keeping. Starting with the introduction of the Census in 1801, through to the registration of births, marriages and deaths later the same century, historians and genealogists can trace with relative ease the whereabouts and circumstances of their ancestors. These sources are used regularly but other records, which are less commonly accessed in terms of research but are actually more revealing, are asylum and poor law records. These unique records ameliorate the information provided from census, birth, marriage and death records and allow a fuller understanding of individuals and their families. Newspaper reports and other sources can help to augment this further. A combination of all these records offers a far greater awareness of these people's mortal existence, their way of life, the hardships they endured, and the circumstances of their death.

Due to the social stigma attached to mental illness, these people are largely forgotten even by their own families. Relatives regularly concealed the details of what they considered to be shameful, and many disorders, which today are either accepted or curable, would be hidden away and not spoken of. In effect, all trace of their identity within the family is removed.

This book will help people explore these records and enable them to understand their significance in a nineteenth century context. Using original documentation, the identities, backgrounds and outcomes for asylum patients will be reconstructed and explored in an attempt to discover their identities in greater detail. In many cases this research leads to a fuller appreciation of their family and the relationships within it.

This book will also explore the medical and social understanding of mental health disorders and the methods used by nineteenth century doctors attempting to cure them. Epilepsy, general paralysis and puerperal insanity are looked at in depth alongside mania, melancholia, dementia and congenital conditions. Nineteenth century case studies are used to illustrate each disorder.

The need for lunatic asylums declined during the twentieth century as care for those with chronic mental illness was transferred to community based psychiatric provision. There are differing views on the development of institutional care in Britain and researchers from a variety of different backgrounds have studied the subject. Some lament the abandoned, derided and deserted asylums, which accommodated isolated communities where the afflicted were cared for, sustained and supported away from the stigmatising view of the general public. Others view the demise of the asylum as a progressive move forward from what many consider was a 'disaster for the insane'.

As nineteenth century lunatic asylums were built to resemble palaces in spacious grounds, many of the buildings are listed as being of historical or architectural significance and therefore are protected. In the majority of cases they have been reused, either as hospitals or as luxury residential houses and apartments. The unique water towers, which many constructed to hold the vast quantities of water needed for daily use, often remain as the only reminder of the building's original use.

Chapter 1

Lunatic Ancestors

Family history is an exciting, compulsive, infectious and fascinating pastime. Many people interested in their own family history will have compiled a basic genealogy with a timeline of their forebears. For most, gathering this list of historical events is a relatively straightforward exercise with each generation having a reliable and valuable set of records to account for the relevant vital events (details of birth, marriage and death). For others, however, an individual may randomly disappear from the usual sources leaving their whereabouts unaccounted for. Emigration to a different country is one possible explanation, as is admission to a hospital, workhouse, or place of learning. However, there is also the chance that an ancestor may have suffered from a mental illness and could have been committed to a lunatic asylum.

Hundreds of thousands of individuals passed through the doors of Victorian lunatic asylums. Many recovered from their illnesses and others were 'relieved' into the care of their relatives or friends. This episode was likely to have been 'brushed under the carpet', but for immediate family members was rarely forgotten due to the negative impact and stigma attached to insanity.

However, many others with mental instability were incarcerated for life and eventually died within these lunatic asylums. More commonly than not, their bodies were never recovered by their relatives – ashamed by, and reluctant to accept, their non-physical illness. Consequently, many families unknowingly have ancestors who experienced asylum life and genealogy is a powerful tool for uncovering a well-kept family secret.

In nineteenth century Britain and Ireland most children were baptised into one of the recognised faiths. The records of these baptisms place that child within their family setting and such details normally give particulars of the date and place of birth and baptism, the names of their parents, their residence, and often their father's occupation. Prior to 1837, in England

and Wales, it was only churches that recorded baptisms, marriages and burial information.

Statutory civil registration of births, marriages and deaths became compulsory in England and Wales on 1 July 1837, on 1 January 1855 in Scotland and on 1 January 1864 in Ireland. This made it a legal requirement to register these vital events within the Registration District in which they took place. The new registrars were required to register all births and deaths in their district. They were paid for each registration and so had an incentive to record as many as possible. However, some births, marriages and deaths inevitably remained unrecorded, particularly in more remote rural areas, and it is estimated that in England and Wales, ten per cent of births were not registered until the law changed in 1874. From that time, parents became legally responsible for informing the registrar of a birth. A similar if not higher statistic also applied to Ireland in the early years of registration. The *Scottish Registration Act* was more rigorously enforced than the early civil registration in England, Wales and Ireland and as a result birth records there are more accurate. In Scotland, parents were required to register a child's birth within twenty-one days. If information was not received after a period of three months, the parents would be subject to a fine of two pounds. As a safeguard, ministers were obliged to inform the registrar if any baby was brought for baptism without an extract of the birth registration being displayed.

A baptismal or birth certificate from the nineteenth century therefore provides the initial piece of documentary evidence to place an individual within their family. Genealogists would next seek census records. The decennial censuses were a count of all people and households and were carried out in England, Wales and Scotland every ten years from 1801 onwards, and in Ireland from 1821. For the majority of places, the 1841 census is the earliest one that records the names of people. Unfortunately, the Irish census records from 1821 to 1851 were destroyed in a fire at the Public Record Office of Ireland in 1922, and the census records from 1861 to 1891 were destroyed by order of the government prior to 1922. The earliest surviving comprehensive Irish census returns are those of 1901 and 1911. The National Archives of Ireland has made these records available online free of charge.

The census provides fairly basic information and gives a list of names of people living in the same household on a given date. The 1841 census does not give an indication of how individuals in a household were related to each other, and adult ages were rounded down to the nearest five which provides an approximate year of birth but cannot be considered accurate. Later census returns became more sophisticated and the latest one available, 1911, provides fairly detailed information about the occupants of a household including details of the size of the property they were living in. This census also recorded how many children had been born to a married couple and how many of them had died. This piece of information is invaluable to researchers as it shows the number of children there would have been in a family and helps account for those who are missing.

Importantly for researchers, some details of sensory and intellectual disability were recorded in the decennial censuses from 1871 onwards, and include whether the individual was (a) Deaf-and-dumb; (b) Blind; (c) Imbecile or Idiot; or (d) Lunatic. It is very unusual to see someone living within a family home listed as a lunatic, although there are exceptions to this, particularly if individuals were boarded out by their parish of origin for a fee. The most notable example of this comes from the village of Kennoway in Fife. The 1891 census return shows that on 5 April 1891, eighteen out of the sixty-eight households in the village boarded imbeciles or lunatics. It records thirty-five imbeciles and two lunatics living with local families.

Due to the perceived stigma, few parents were likely to acknowledge lunacy in an offspring – many at that time believed that lunacy was inherited. Imbecility and idiocy seemed more acceptable especially if the defect was present at birth, and there are occasions where this is listed for an individual living with their family. Lunatic, however, is a term that is generally only seen on asylum, hospital or workhouse census returns.

Name and surname	Position in the institution	Condition as to marriage	Age	Profession or occupation	Where born	Disability
S.L.	Patient	Single	23	Servant Domestic	Russia	Lunatic
S.L.	ditto	Single	71		England	Blind
A.E.L.	ditto	Married	53	Plain needlework	Suffolk	Lunatic

Extract from 1901 census for Colney Hatch, London County Lunatic Asylum.

Name and surname	Position in the institution	Condition as to marriage	Age	Profession or occupation	Where born	Disability
Thomas Cowan	Patient	Single	24	General labourer	Not recorded	Imbecile
Leonard L. Cookson	ditto	Single	29	Painter	Derbyshire	Lunatic
George A. Clarke	ditto	Married	38	Engineer	Middlesex	Lunatic

Extract from 1901 census for Cheshire County Lunatic Asylum, Upton, Chester.

Many, but not all, asylums concealed the identity of their patients on the census, referring to them only by their initials.

The Lunacy Commission in England and Wales kept registers from 1846 of patients in both public and private asylums. These record the name, age and gender of the patient; the name of hospital, asylum, or licensed madhouse; and the date of their admission, discharge or death. These registers are available at the National Archives at Kew and online via several subscription websites. Therefore, if lack of information on a census fails to show the presence of a family member in an asylum, the Lunacy Registers are worth researching.

Central registers were also kept for the Scottish asylums. Mental Welfare Commission records consisting of Notices of Admissions by the Superintendent of the Mental Institutions 1858–1962 and General Register of Lunatics in Asylums 1805–1978 are not available online but are held at The National Records of Scotland.

The Scottish General Register of Lunatics in Asylums from 1805 is a chronological list of names of patients giving details of their date of admission, discharge or death, and observations of their condition in the asylum. The register also provides information regarding whose care the patient was in and the parochial board responsible for funding the admission. The Admission Books are a series of monthly volumes dating from 1858 that contain bound copies of the Notices of Admissions by the superintendent of the mental institutions addressed to the Secretary of the Board. The Notices of Admission contains a report on the patient by the admitting physician, details of the petition to the Sheriff, personal details of the patient, two medical certificates and an emergency order granted by the Sheriff. The type of personal information contained in these volumes includes name, age, marital status, religion, place of residence, age and duration of first attack with other medical information for each patient. The Notice of Admittance gives the name of the asylum each patient was sent to.

Researching a family using medical case notes provides a wealth of rich and detailed information that is not obtainable from other sources. The facts provided in these records are of a sensitive nature and are correctly unavailable to researchers for 100 years after the date of recording due to ethical, confidentiality and privacy considerations. However, they may provide a far clearer picture of family life and the facts are given directly by either the patient themselves, their next of kin, or a representative speaking on their behalf who knew them well. Medical case notes provide background details of patients on admission and chronicle their stay at the asylum. Information regarding their 'friends' who are generally a family member are provided, as are details of hereditary illness if known. An address for the patient prior to admission is provided although on occasions this may be the union workhouse, parochial poorhouse or another asylum if they had been transferred. The union or parish responsible for the payment of asylum fees is provided on the documentation but, as can be seen from the census extracts above, this is not necessarily the place a patient was born. The medical case notes in England and Wales do not show a date or place of birth for patients, nor in many cases parental details; in the case of married women, maiden surnames are not always provided. Similar information is contained within Scottish and Irish records with many asylums providing fuller particulars as the century progressed.

Few genealogical sources provide such full, detailed and occasionally private information. Even for patients who were only admitted for short periods of time, asylum records provide details about why the admission was necessary and the outcome of their stay in the asylum. However, there is also often information about their extended family that would not be obtainable from other sources. This may include not only the names of relatives, but also details of the interaction, family dynamics and personalities of other family members through the eyes of the asylum staff and the patients themselves. There may be information regarding the state of health, if alive, of parents and grandparents, or otherwise their cause

14

of death. Hereditary diseases in the family, especially mental disorders, are often recorded.

Case study: Janet Fernie

Janet Fernie was a 28-year-old married domestic servant admitted to the Roxburgh, Berwick and Selkirk District Lunatic Asylum with acute mania in December 1889. The admission notes record that she was the wife of a wheelwright and had been married for eight years. They make reference to her four children but do not name them and her husband is similarly unnamed. The notes do state, however, that 'her father's sister's daughter is a patient here, Isabella Hope, case number 988.' Janet's father is named as Thomas Huggan, a joiner at St Mary's, Dingleton, Melrose.

Matching the asylum records to those of Poor Law applications, far greater information is revealed about her family with her admission to the asylum being recorded on 21 December 1889. Details of her husband, her parents and the various family residences are given. She was the wife of Alexander Fernie, a wheelwright, employed at Aberfeldy, Perthshire. Her parents are named as Thomas Huggan and Mary Holmes. Her six addresses over a seven year period are provided, as are the names and ages of all four children.

This corroborative information provides a clear picture of a family unit over nearly a decade and brings together evidence of their lives that would not be obtainable from other sources.

Case studies: Esther and Violet Gosling

Sisters Esther and Violet Gosling died in their early twenties in the late 1890s. The death certificate for each sister gave the cause of death as 'epilepsy'. Neither sister had died in an asylum, but epilepsy was considered incurable in the nineteenth century and many individuals who suffered from seizures were sent to asylums. Asylum admission registers were consulted to determine if either sister had been admitted for her disability. These revealed that both sisters had been admitted to the same asylum on the same day and had later been relieved to the care of their family. Discovering this information allowed for a more thorough examination of the case notes for the sisters at the relevant record office. There was a full description of their condition, photographs of both sisters and details that epilepsy was hereditary in the family. This allowed further research to take place to determine who else in the family suffered with the same condition. It was later discovered that their paternal uncle, Moses Gosling, had also been in an asylum suffering from epilepsy.

Another source of information indicating that an ancestor had been in an asylum is the registration of a death; death certificates show where and when people died. If they died in an asylum, this is stated on the certificate and the entry will also indicate whether a post-mortem or inquest took place following the death. Some asylums routinely carried out post-mortems even when the cause of death was obvious to the asylum doctors. Armed with this knowledge, a visit to the relevant record office should enable research within the patient case books.

Case study: Sarah Swindells

Sarah Swindells was a 32-year-old domestic servant living at Stockport, Cheshire. She was admitted to Parkside Asylum in Macclesfield, Cheshire on 12 May 1880 and diagnosed with epileptic insanity. Prior to this she had been in Stockport Union Workhouse because she had tried to commit suicide by jumping out of a window.

She was initially described as having no signs of active insanity and was a very useful and helpful patient – willing and able to scrub floors all day if necessary. She remained fit and well for over two years, had occasional epileptic seizures, generally at night, and expressed a desire to return home saying she felt quite well. Her epilepsy increased suddenly and without apparent warning. In July 1883 she had successive seizures over a period of two days before falling into a comatose state. She died without regaining consciousness. Despite having been continually monitored by asylum staff during her last days, a post-mortem was conducted to establish her cause of death and confirmed that she had died of epilepsy.

Notices of death issued by the asylum for patients were more detailed than the civil registration certificates recorded in the General Register Office in England and Wales. The asylum notices provide details of admission dates to the asylum and the supposed cause of insanity together with the assumed cause of death. They also include the time of death and record which member(s) of staff were in attendance. Information about mechanical restraint is also reported if it had been used on the patient within seven days of their demise.

Depending on which asylum individuals were admitted to, the extent of available records will vary. In some cases no records have survived. There are however very complete records for many counties – records that will enhance understanding of a family. Typical patient records available are likely to consist of the following for England and Wales:

Asylum Pauper and Private Admission Registers

Typically, asylum admission registers contain the name, age and sex of patients; the date of their admission; the form of mental disorder they had and its duration; their union of origin and, where applicable, their address; and details concerning the outcome of the admission which would be 'recovered', 'relieved', 'transferred' or 'died'.

Asylum Medical Case Notes

Medical case notes provide background details of patients on admission and chronicle their stay at the asylum. Information regarding their 'friends' (who are generally family members are provided), as are details of hereditary illness if known. An address for the patient prior to admission is provided although on occasions this is the union workhouse or another asylum if they had been transferred. There is no date or place of birth of patients, nor in many cases parental details; in the case of married women, maiden surnames are rarely provided.

Case notes occasionally allow for the patient's voice to be 'heard' alongside those caring for them prior and during admission. There are often photographs on admission and on discharge and detailed information regarding the medical treatment they received. Death information is included as is a copy of the death certificate.

Asylum Register of Discharges, Removals and Deaths

For those who died in the asylum, these registers provide the exact date of death. Details of deaths are also obtainable through patient case notes. However, due to the 100 year closure rule for medical records, patients who died less than 100 years ago are only available in the above register. These registers also include details of discharges and removals from the asylum.

Medical Superintendent's Letter Book

This volume contains copies of the Medical Superintendent's reports to the Commissioner of Lunacy detailing the reasons why each patient was admitted to the asylum. A statement regarding a patient's physical and mental health was also noted.

Mechanical Restraint Register

Following the 1890 *Lunacy Act* it became a legal requirement for asylums to keep a register of patients who had been mechanically restrained in any way. This register may include information such as the use of mittens to prevent scratching or induce vomiting, jackets or dresses made of strong linen to prevent them being torn, laced or buttoned at the back with long sleeves fastened to the dress at the shoulders with closed ends for tying behind the back when the arms had been folded across the chest. Sheets or towels could be used to fasten patients into their beds or chairs to prevent excessive movement. The reason for the use of such items was noted in the register.

Workhouse Admissions, Discharges and Creed Registers

For individuals who were admitted to an asylum from the workhouse, it is useful to check the above registers which should provide additional information on the circumstances they found themselves in to be in need of parish care. The Creed Registers in particular are extremely useful as they provide details of names, date of birth, date and place of admission, religious creed, the source of the information and date of discharge or death. Additionally, some creed registers provide the occupation, last address and name and address of an individual's nearest relative.

Similar records were kept for the Scottish and Irish equivalents of workhouses. They were termed 'poorhouses' in Scotland and 'houses of industry' in Ireland.

Medical case notes are therefore an excellent way of understanding more about members of a family and, as such, are useful additions for any researcher. In order to understand the laws that governed the incarceration of the mentally ill and the need for the expansion of the asylum system, the following chapters reveal why changes took place and what impact they had on those who were described as 'idiots', 'imbeciles' and lunatics in nineteenth century Great Britain and Ireland.

As asylums grew in size so did the number of staff employed within them. It is possible to track not only a patient journey through an asylum but also the staff that worked there. Asylum staff are mentioned by job title and occasionally by name throughout patient case notes. Members of staff who were with patients when they died are always referred to by name on the subsequent death certificate. As a result, it is worth consulting asylum documentation as a record of their employment.

Case study: William Wilson
On 18 December 1869, two asylum attendants, Samuel Robert Wood and John Hodgson killed a patient in their charge: William Wilson, a 54-year-old former innkeeper who had been committed to Lancaster asylum three days before his death. At a coroner's inquest on 29 December 1869, both Wood and Hodgson were found guilty of causing the death of the patient William Wilson and were committed for trial at Lancaster assizes. The following article from the *Manchester Courier* details the Coroner's inquest.

William Wilson, innkeeper of Butsbeck near Dalton.

The Coroner's inquest [29 December 1869]
The death from violence in Lancaster Asylum
Committal of two Attendants for Manslaughter.

The inquiry into the circumstances attending the death of William Wilson, a patient in Lancaster Lunatic Asylum, who died on the 26th instant from the effects of twelve broken ribs, was resumed at the asylum on Wednesday afternoon. The medical evidence on the previous day showed that deceased died of pleurisy, brought on by the fracture of twelve of his ribs, six on each side. The attendants who had charge of the deceased from the date of his admission, on the 15th inst., up to the time the injuries were discovered, all swore that they used no violence towards him, and that they were not aware violence had been used by any other person. On Wednesday, a patient named James Dutton – a remarkably intelligent witness – was sworn, and gave important evidence. He came from Liverpool, and was a fireman on a steam boat. He knew the patient who was hurt, and saw two of the attendants ill-use him. He thought it was on Saturday 18th, but could not speak with certainty. One of the attendants who abused the deceased was named Wood, the other was 'the tallest of the attendants in No 1 Ward,' he did not know his name. The tall attendant 'struck deceased several times, and kicked him too, and knocked him down, and kicked him while he was lying on the ground, and then left him.' The 'tall attendant' then left the room. Witness afterwards heard an attendant named Wood say the deceased man had hit him on the nose, and tell him (the deceased) to 'wait till my nose gives over bleeding, and then see what I'll do for you.' Witness was persuading deceased not to interfere, and to be quiet, or he 'would get ill-used,' when Wood went towards where they were sitting, got hold of the old gentleman (meaning the deceased), pulled him onto the boards, and kicked him in different parts of the body. Wood then took deceased by the collar, till he was red in the face and afterwards witness saw him jerk his knees into different parts of the deceased's body while he was lying upon the floor. There were a great many patients in the ward at the time this violence was said to have been committed, but the medical officers of the asylum did not consider them capable of giving evidence. The witness Dutton identified the attendant John Hodgson as the 'tall attendant' he had referred to in his evidence.

The jury were four hours in deciding upon the terms of their verdict, and they ultimately found 'That the deceased died of the injuries he received, and that those injuries were inflicted by Samuel Wood and John Hodgson.' The Coroner said he should take this as a verdict of manslaughter against the two attendants, and they were committed for trial at the assizes. The deceased was 54 years of age.

Manchester Courier, 31 December 1869

The Attendants

Wood and Hodgson were brought before the Lancashire magistrates on 12 January 1870 on a charge of wilful murder. The bench committed both men for trial, which led to their conviction of manslaughter in March 1870. They were both tried for killing and slaying William Wilson, but Wood was also tried with the additional offence of 'malice aforethought'. They both received a sentence of seven years' penal servitude.

John Hodgson was 24 years old, newly married and his young wife was pregnant with their first child when he was sent to pick oakum at Lancaster Prison at the beginning of his sentence. Within two months he was transferred to HM Prison Pentonville in London where he remained

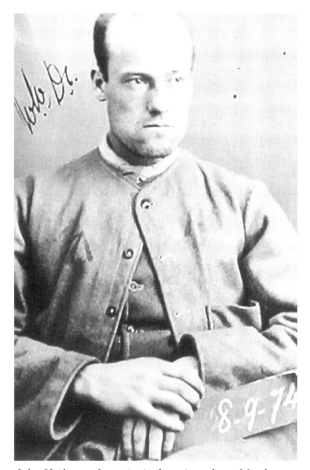

John Hodgson, Lunatic Asylum Attendant; Murderer.

for five months before being transferred to Woking Invalid Convict Prison for the remainder of his sentence. Woking was the first prison specifically built for disabled prisoners – not just for the physically ill, but also those suffering from mental illness. There is no suggestion from the prison records that John was physically unwell – on the contrary, his health was described as good and his physique tall and strong on his release. He returned to his wife and 5-year-old son, John, in Lancaster on licence on 14 August 1875. The couple remained in Lancashire and had three more children. John remained out of prison and asylums for the rest of his life.

Samuel Robert Wood was convicted on the more serious charge of manslaughter with malice aforethought but received the same sentence of seven years' penal servitude as John Hodgson. He was a 24-year-old single man, the son of John Wood, a shoemaker from Lancaster. Like Hodgson, Wood began his sentence picking oakum at Lancaster before being transferred to HM Prison Pentonville in May 1870. He served the majority of his sentence at HM Prison Portsmouth and HM Prison Portland before being released on licence on 9 August 1875. The prison records show that his parents and siblings moved away from Lancaster after his imprisonment but they remained in contact with him for the duration of his sentence. On his release he went to live with his elderly mother Thomasine in Burnley, Lancashire, where he earned a living from giving music lessons and tuning pianos.

Their victim
William Wilson was a 54-year-old innkeeper from The Bridge Inn, Batsbeck, Dalton in Furness. He was admitted to Lancaster asylum on 15 December 1869 and diagnosed with General Paralysis of the Insane (see Chapter 15 for further details). Three days later he was beaten so badly by Wood and Hodgson that he suffered twelve broken ribs and died on 26 December 1869 from pleurisy.

The remarkably intelligent witness
A witness to the crime was called to give evidence at the coroner's court and at the trial at Lancaster assizes. Described as 'a remarkably intelligent witness', James Dutton was an asylum inmate who shared a ward with William Wilson. Originating from Liverpool and having previously been a fireman on a steam boat, Dutton had been in the asylum since 16 February 1869. He died there on 28 May 1886.

Not every asylum attendant mistreated their patients; the majority were caring individuals dedicated to the nursing of the insane. For more information on asylum attendants and other asylum staff see Chapter 11.

New asylum regulations in the nineteenth century sought to provide a sheltered and caring environment for patients, and staff were accountable for their actions, treatment and care of the insane. This had not been the case in previous centuries when barbaric practises and the ridicule of those afflicted with mental health disorders was the norm.

Chapter 2

The Pre-Nineteenth Century Setting

The treatment of the mentally ill in Great Britain and Ireland before the nineteenth century was nothing short of cruel. Pre-conceived ideas about the nature of 'madness' and the lack of any rational medical understanding of its many manifestations meant that sufferers could become victims of derision, ridicule and even neglect. During the eighteenth century people had diverse opinions regarding madness – fearful of its close proximity and suddenness of attack yet, at the same time, fascinated and captivated by the bizarre behaviours of the mentally ill.

England and Wales

Bethlehem (Bethlem) Royal Hospital in London had been established as early as the mid-thirteenth century as the Priory of the New Order of St Mary of Bethlem in Bishopgate, London. It was not initially intended as a refuge for the mentally ill, but rather a priory that housed the poor and offered hospitality for visiting clergy. Its use and location changed over time and by the fourteenth century, it had begun to specialise in the care and control of the insane. Its name changed colloquially over time to 'Bedlam' and the word itself became synonymous with madness and continues to be used today to signify chaos and irrationality.

Chains, manacles and stocks were widely used to control the 'furious' inmates. A committee appointed in 1598 declared the house to be so loathsome and dirty that it was not fit for any man to enter. Due to an increase in the number of patients, the initial building at Bishopgate became too small, and a larger, more lavish and luxurious institution, 'New Bethlem', was built at huge expense at Moorfields in London opening in 1676.

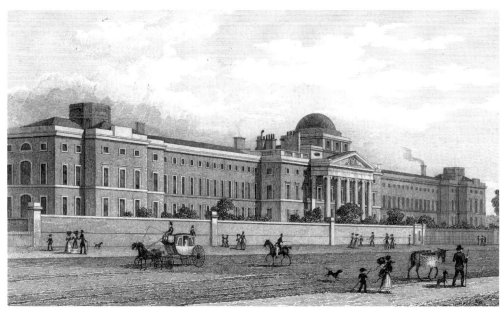

London Old Bethlem Hospital at Moorfields in about 1750 - Antique Print 1892.

The asylum moved again in 1815 to a new, more substantial Bethlem Asylum at St George's Fields at Lambeth. A further move to Monks Orchard at Addington, Surrey, in 1930 helped once again to improve patient conditions. Although this site was further away from the city, it provided patients with more space for indoor and outdoor activities. The former Bethlem buildings in Lambeth were subsequently purchased by Lord Rothermere in 1930 and were developed into the Imperial War Museum.

The first piece of legislation concerning the safe custody of individuals with mental health disorders was introduced in 1714 with the *Vagrancy Act*. The Act stated that:

> *there are sometimes in parishes, towns and places, persons of little or no estates, who, by lunacy, or otherwise, are furiously mad, and dangerous to be permitted to go abroad, ... that it shall and may be lawful for any two or more of the Justices of the Peace of any county, town or place in England, Wales or Town of Berwick upon Tweed, where such lunatic or mad person shall be found, by warrant under their hands and seals, directed to the*

24

constables, church-wardens, and overseers of the poor of such parish, town or place, or some of them, to cause such person to be apprehended.

However, whilst this legislation allowed those deemed to be insane to be removed from society, it did not safeguard them from the institutions in which they were incarcerated. An amended *Vagrancy Act* of 1744 allowed local authorities to board out the detained lunatics in private madhouses. It was not until the introduction of the *Madhouse Act* of 1774 that the Royal College of Physicians were required to monitor and license madhouses in order to protect the patients contained within them. The Act stated that:

many great and dangerous abuses arose from the present state of houses kept for the reception of lunatics, for want of regulations with respect to the persons keeping such houses, the admission of patients into them and the visitation by proper persons of the said houses and patients: and whereas the law, as it now stands, is insufficient for preventing or discovering such abuses.

In theory this act should have safeguarded and protected those incarcerated in asylums. However, as will be seen, it was not until 1815 that the full horrors of asylum life were revealed.

During the seventeenth and eighteenth century it became practise for the educated, wealthy and well-bred of London to 'visit' Bethlem Asylum in much the same way that they may have visited a zoo or theatre – for their own amusement and as a way of ridiculing the poor, half-starved individuals raving in chains and lying in their own excrement. This custom was encouraged by the asylum Governors because it provided additional revenue in the form of two-pence admission fees, donations and legacies intended for the benefit of the poor inmates. In many cases the money enriched the pockets of those in charge. This practise was essentially stopped in 1770 when visitors were required to have a ticket signed by the Governor. Whilst the patients were undoubtedly seen as figures of fun and amusement for the entertainment of visitors, the presence of outsiders prevented the asylum staff from committing abuses on them. It is thought that patient mistreatment may well have escalated as a result of the asylum becoming a closed, unregulated community in

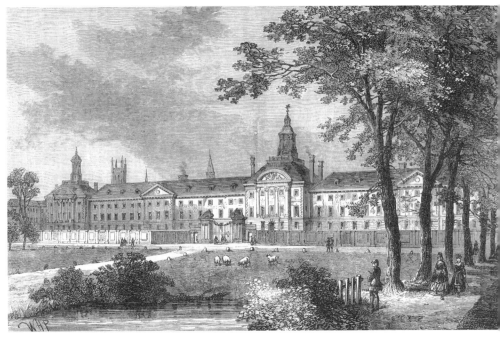

New Bethlem Hospital, St George's Fields (now the Imperial War Museum). Steel Engraving. Drawn by Thomas H. Shepherd. Engraved by J. Tingle, 1830.

the late eighteenth century. While visits from spectators were welcomed for the revenue it brought to the asylum, visits from medical practitioners and the clergy were not encouraged.

Bethlem Asylum was very much 'a family affair' managed and administered by the Monro family for four generations between 1728 and 1853. The first of this family, James Monro (1680–1752), was almost the only doctor in London during the eighteenth century who 'specialised' in the cure of the mind, although Bethlem was not the only asylum claiming to be able to cure conditions relating to mental health. There were many private madhouses throughout the country including at least two in London owned by the same Monro family who were in charge at Bethlem. There were also wards for lunatics in several of the London hospitals.

At the beginning of the nineteenth century, the Bethlem apothecary was John Haslam (1764–1844) who had trained at the United Borough Hospitals in London and in Edinburgh. He was awarded an MD by the University of Aberdeen in 1816. He appears to have been an energetic and intelligent man greatly interested in 'the state of the brain' and 'its consistence in maniacal disorders'. However, Haslam was less concerned with the living conditions of the patients of the asylum and more concerned with the nature of their madness, which he attempted to prove as a result of post-mortem examinations.

A Select Committee enquiry was conducted in 1815 to consider the better Regulation of Madhouses, in England. One of the reasons for this enquiry was due to the visit to Bethlem in 1814 of the Member of Parliament and Quaker philanthropist Edward Wakefield and the resulting scandals that were exposed about the way patients were being treated. Despite the difficulties the committee initially had at gaining entry, the following is an extract from the findings of Edward Wakefield's visit:

At this first visit, attended by the steward of the Hospital and likewise by a female keeper, we first proceeded to visit the women's galleries: one of the side rooms contained about ten patients, each chained by one arm or leg to the wall; the chain allowing them merely to stand up by the bench or form fixed to the wall, or to sit down on it. The nakedness of each patient was covered by a blanket-gown only; the blanket-gown is a blanket formed something like a dressing-gown, with nothing to fasten it with in front; this constitutes the whole covering; the feet even were naked. One female in this side room, thus chained, was an object remarkably striking; she mentioned her maiden and married names, and stated that she had been a teacher of languages; the keepers described her as a very accomplished lady, mistress of many languages, and corroborated her account of herself. The Committee can hardly imagine a human being in a more degraded and brutalizing situation than that in which I found this female, who held a coherent conversation with us, and was of course fully sensible of the mental and bodily condition of those wretched beings, who, equally without clothing, were closely chained to the same wall with herself.

John Haslam, the apothecary, and Thomas Monro, the physician, both lost their posts as a result of the findings. Thomas Monro's only explanation to the committee regarding the conditions his patients were living in was that 'it was handed down to me by my father, and I do not know any better practise.' Bethlem was not the only asylum reviewed by the Select Committee and others throughout the country were also visited and found to have patients living in similar conditions.

Following a visit to St Peter's at Bristol, the committee deemed it to be totally unfit for an asylum and recommended that the entire body of lunatics ought to be moved to more spacious premises and to a more healthy and airy situation. Their report from St Peter's contains the following description:

> *The part of the Bristol Workhouse called St. Peter's Hospital, set apart for the Pauper Lunatics of the city, is without any day-room, eating-room or kitchen for the females distinct from their sleeping apartments; and the only place in which they (40 in number) can take exercise is a small passage or paved yard at one end of the Hospital. It is part of the road for carts to the Workhouse, and measures about 37 feet by 18, and is, from its pavement and extent utterly unfit for an airing-ground. The yard, very little larger than that appropriated to the Females. There are small wooden closets, or Pens, for confining the violent and refractory Patients. Those for the men were 7 feet long by 3 feet 3 inches broad and about 9 feet high, and were warmed by pipes, and a hole in the door, and also a hole in the ceiling for ventilation. The Pens for the Women were smaller and were not warmed, and were ill ventilated. The walls of each were of wood, but were not padded. Formerly, Patients were occasionally kept in those Pens during both day and night, but the Pens are now very rarely used. In addition to the jacket and leg-locks, a sort of open mask of leather passing round the face, and also round the forehead to the back of the head, and fastened by leather straps, was at one time placed over the heads of such Patients as were in the habit of biting; but this mask (as the Commissioners understand) has been for some time discontinued.*

The asylum at York was also investigated by a local magistrate following allegations of cruelty, abuse, and embezzlement. Mysteriously, in December 1813, the asylum burnt down killing four patients and destroying all records before an official enquiry could be started.

While the main focus of the enquiry was Bethlem and York, the committee aimed to discover the truth about patient care and conditions in as many asylums, madhouses and workhouses as possible. As well as making some horrific discoveries, their reports also contain impressive accounts of excellent practise and management. The evidence gathered by the Select Committee enabled the public to view insanity in a different light for the first time. Instead of encouraging people to ridicule and visit for amusement there was a definite shift towards the regulation and reform of asylums. Legislation regulating the care of the mentally ill did not change for a further thirteen years.

As the Select Committee discovered, not all asylums at the beginning of the nineteenth century employed methods of restraint. A pioneering group of alienists or 'mad doctors' opened asylums that relied instead on moral therapy for the care and cure of patients. A visit to a friend Hannah Mills, a Quaker from Leeds, who later died in the asylum at York in April 1790 aroused William Tuke's (1732–1822) suspicions that she had not received good care and treatment. As at Bethlem, friends attempting to visit relatives at the York asylum had been prevented from doing so even

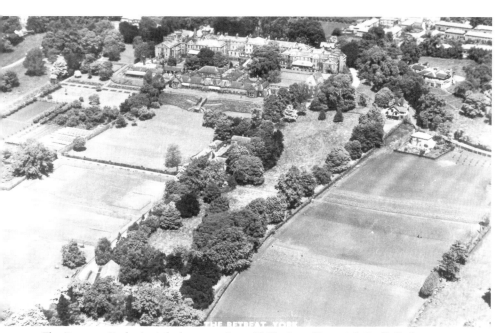

The Retreat, York. Aerial photograph. c. 1960. Aero Pictorial, Redhill, Surrey.

when patients had requested religious guidance and support. In 1792, the York Retreat was set up by William Tuke who, like Edward Wakefield, was a Quaker. The York Retreat was one of the first establishments in Great Britain and Ireland to treat patients as human beings and offer a therapeutic setting for them. Mechanical restraints were discontinued and work and leisure became the main treatment. This use of kindness and care as a way of helping patients recover from their disorders became known as 'moral therapy'. The belief that kindness cured, and ill-treatment exacerbated mental health disorders, was revolutionary at this time.

An extract passing the resolution from the Society of Friends in York stated that:

ground be purchased, and a building be erected sufficient to accommodate thirty patients, in an airy situation, and at as short a distance from York as may be, so as to have the privilege of retirement; and that there be a few acres for keeping cows, and for garden ground for the family, which will afford scope for the patients to take exercise when that may be prudent and suitable.

William Tuke gave evidence to the Select Committee in 1815 about conditions in other asylums and his methods of treatment at The Retreat gained him an unrivalled reputation in the therapeutic care of the insane. Without doubt his philosophy concerning the care of the mentally ill was forward thinking for its time and was not necessarily accepted by all, many of whom still believed in the use of mechanical restraint to manage mental health instead of calm and kindness. Tuke is credited for setting in motion a system that would eventually be adopted at parliamentary level for the future provision of the insane.

State funded asylums were rare before the nineteenth century and there were few hospitals able to cater for the mentally ill. As a result, many individuals considered to be insane were left within their communities, often ending up in either workhouses or gaols. Whilst it had been common practise in England and Wales to restrain lunatic patients in asylums, newspaper reports from the period also reveal the harsh treatment the insane received within their family homes. The stigma attached to having mentally ill relatives meant many were kept hidden away from public gaze. In December 1818, husband and wife Charles and Leonora Elliott were tried at the Middlesex Sessions and found guilty of cruelty to their

9 year old son who was tied naked to his bed by a leather strap, fed irregularly on bread and water, and hidden from view from neighbours. The couple declared that it would have cost them as much as three shillings a week to send their son to the workhouse to be cared for and they needed the money to care for themselves and their other children. Both husband and wife were sentenced to terms of imprisonment by the court.

A requirement for legislation that would provide a place of refuge and care for the mentally ill was desperately needed and a campaign set in motion changes that would help those deemed to be insane.

Scotland

In Scotland, provision for individuals with mental health disorders was recognised in law as early as the fourteenth century when a statute of Robert the Bruce, King Robert I of Scotland, placed the responsibility for the upkeep and custody of persons of 'furious mind' upon their relatives, and failing them on the Sheriff of the county in which they lived.

Two types of lunatic were defined in Scotland at that time – the 'fatuous' and the 'furious'. The fatuous, or imbecilic, lunatic could be committed into the custody of the next agnate – the 'nearest male relative on the father's side', whereas the custody of the furious or 'raving mad' lunatic belonged to the Crown 'as having the sole power of coercing them with fetters'.

In the eighteenth and early-nineteenth centuries, 'lunatics' were frequently placed in rather basic, scant and inappropriate accommodation. To a large extent, what happened when an individual became insane depended on his position in society. If he was of independent means, his nearest relative was responsible for taking the necessary steps to place him in an appropriate madhouse. If he was a pauper, the inspector of poor for his parish acted on his behalf. If he was dangerous, the Procurator Fiscal, on behalf of the public, had the legal duty of placing him under care. In all cases, a medical certificate of insanity was required. A petition was then made to the Sheriff to grant a warrant for committal to an asylum or other suitable place.

Pauper lunatics were defined as 'lunatics, who, not having adequate means of support, are chargeable on poor-rates'. They were looked after by family, neighbours and communities with varying degrees of care. Insane paupers who were not cared for by their families at home, perhaps because there was no close surviving relative to tend to them, could be incarcerated by their parish inspector of poor without a warrant in gaols, prisons, poorhouses or in private licensed 'madhouses'. They could also be confined indefinitely in hospitals. Many harmless 'half-wits' were left to their own devices and were allowed to roam freely, or 'at large' around the countryside.

Up until 1781 there was only one lunatic hospital in Scotland – the Edinburgh Bedlam, or Darien House Hospital, built in 1698 in Greyfriars Yard. The ruling class Scots were very generous, particularly to one another. Through their philanthropic endowments by way of legacies, subscriptions and donations, improvements in mental care provision for the well-to-do escalated. Seven 'Royal', otherwise known as 'chartered', asylums were established throughout Scotland in the late-eighteenth and early-nineteenth centuries, set up as charitable foundations. Private patients suffering from mental disorders who had the means to pay, could be admitted to one of these seven luxurious asylums, paying between £30 and £300 a year depending on the amenities provided. These asylums resembled large, upper class country houses and were situated in elevated, salubrious locations. The residents were properly provided for in spacious, comfortable and well-appointed accommodation. Founded in 1781, Sunnyside Royal Hospital at Montrose was the first of these to open. Sunnyside obtained a Royal Charter in 1810 as Montrose Lunatic Asylum, Infirmary & Dispensary.

It was not until after the 1857 *Lunacy (Scotland) Act* that a publicly funded network of pauper lunatic asylums would be established.

Ireland

He gave the little Wealth he had
To build a House for Fools and Mad
And shew'd by one satyric Touch
No Nation wanted it so much.

'Verses on the Death of Dr Swift'; Jonathan Swift, 1731.

The two kingdoms of Great Britain and Ireland united under the Acts of Union in 1801. This political manoeuvre effectively brought Ireland under Westminster rule. Many commentators have suggested that Ireland was subsequently considered by the English to be one of their many colonies.

THE PRE-NINETEENTH CENTURY SETTING

There was no poor law in Ireland at the beginning of the nineteenth century, therefore parishes were not obliged to maintain impoverished lunatics or idiots. Workhouses, termed 'houses of industry', were established in the larger Irish cities of Dublin, Cork, Waterford, Limerick and Clonmel from 1772 onwards as punitive, rather than charitable establishments, to remove the 'undeserving undesirables' from the streets and detain them for up to four years. In his 1799 *Account of the late improvements in the house of industry at Dublin*, the English social reformer Sir Thomas Bernard (1750-1818) commented:

> *It is to be observed, that this institution differs very materially from any poorhouse, or other institution, in Great Britain, both in its object, its government, and its resources. In Ireland there are no poor laws, or local taxes, for the support of the poor. This institution was provided for the purpose of providing employment, and for maintenance of the poor of Dublin, and for the punishment of the vagrants and beggars who infested the streets of that city.*

The original houses of industry accommodated only a few lunatics and idiots who were admitted voluntarily and usually only for short periods of time if they were without means. However, it soon became apparent that there was a need for separate accommodation for lunatics as they could be disruptive to the other inmates and to the routine of the workhouse. Houses of industry started to provide cells for lunatics – ten cells for insane persons were provided in Dublin's house of industry in 1776. The Irish *Prisons Act* of 1787 empowered Grand Juries (the county administrative and judicial bodies) to raise public funds to establish lunatic wards in houses of industry and thus provide specific accommodation for the destitute insane – provided that they had been certified by at least two magistrates.

Until that time there were very few facilities to care for the mentally ill in Ireland – most of those afflicted were looked after by their families or communities, or wandered at large as vagrants. A few were placed in workhouses or prisons. A 'madhouse' had been built in 1711 attached to the infirmary of the Royal Hospital at Kilmainham, Dublin, for soldiers who 'by unaccountable accidents in the service, sometimes happen to become lunatics'. It continued in use until 1849.

The number of insane patients in Ireland grew steadily in the eighteenth century and provision for their care remained in short supply. One of the reasons for their increase in number was an increase in the population, which more than doubled between 1750 and 1790 due to the economic growth and prosperity of the country.

The 1787 *Prisons Act*, passed by the Parliament of Ireland, permitted the Irish Grand Juries – responsible for administration at county level – to raise funds for the establishment of 'houses of industry', for the relief of their poor which should have attached lunatic wards. Gradually, public provision for the insane in Ireland was made by erecting cells in houses of industry. However, by 1800, only four out of the thirty-two counties of Ireland – Dublin, Cork, Waterford and Limerick – had made any provision to care for lunatics in these houses of industry.

Dr William Saunders Hallaran (c.1765–1825), a graduate of the University of Edinburgh and visiting physician to Cork Public Asylum also owned a small private asylum at Blackrock near Cork known as the 'Cittadella' which opened in 1798. At the beginning of the nineteenth century he published '*An Enquiry into the Causes Producing the Extraordinary Addition to the Number of Insane*' which was subsequently republished as '*Practical Observations on the Causes and Cure of Insanity*'. Hallaran declared that 'it was an incontrovertible fact that, from the year 1798 to 1809, the number of insane had advanced far beyond the extent of any former period'. He attributed this to both psychological and medical causes following the terror of the 1798 rebellion and the growing number of heredity cases of insanity.

Hallaran's book and the increase in the numbers of insane ensured that the English authorities acted to enhance the provision for the mentally ill of Ireland. In 1810 they authorised the building of a separate asylum 'for the reception of lunatics from all parts of the Kingdom'. The Richmond Lunatic Asylum, more commonly known as Grangegorman, opened in Dublin in 1815 for 200 patients.

Prior to Grangegorman, the largest establishment in Ireland catering for pauper lunatics was St Patrick's Hospital in Dublin – a charitable institution also known as Swift's Hospital. It was founded in 1747 through a legacy of £11,000 from the writer Jonathan Swift (1667–1745), who was Dean of St Patrick's Cathedral in Dublin from 1713 until his death. Swift had previously been a governor of London's Bedlam Hospital and he bequeathed 'his whole fortune, excepting some legacies, to build and

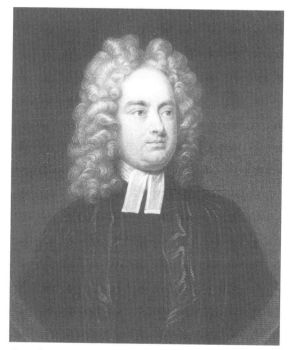

Jonathan Swift. Engraving by B. Holl, 1835.

endow a hospital, in or near this city [Dublin] for the support of idiots, lunaticks, [sic] and those they call incurables'. Swift's Hospital opened in 1757 as St Patrick's Hospital for Imbeciles, initially for fifty fee-paying patients. Pauper patients were admitted from 1776. By 1800, with parliamentary grants, legacies and donations, the hospital had been extended twice and at that time accommodated about 150 lunatic patients.

Despite the population explosion and the grossly inadequate conditions for the provision of care for the mentally ill in Ireland towards the end of the eighteenth century, by the early nineteenth century Sir Andrew Halliday (1782–1839), Royal Physician to William IV and Queen Victoria, remarked that, 'Ireland is the only portion of the British Empire where just views have been entertained of what was necessary for the comfort and cure of her insane population ... Oh that England would be wise, and would consider this, and for once take a lesson from her more humble sister!'

Chapter 3

Lunacy Legislation in Great Britain and Ireland

Legislation in England and Wales

Prior to the reform of the Poor Laws in 1834, the provision of care for the mentally ill in England and Wales lacked legal restrictions and as such many people saw it as a highly profitable field for exploitation. In 1788, the serendipitous circumstances surrounding the mania of the reigning monarch, King George III, ensured that the topic of insanity became widely discussed in both medical and government circles. The revelations achieved by the Select Committee whilst considering their report on madhouses in 1815 also heightened the public's awareness of the stark abuses, ill-treatment and embezzlement committed on those who were most vulnerable.

In England and Wales a new *County Asylums Act* was passed in 1808 requiring the use of public funds to establish places to care for people with mental health problems. The Act stated that 'The practice of confining such lunatics and other insane persons as are chargeable to their respective parishes in Gaols, Houses of Correction, Poor Houses and Houses of Industry, is highly dangerous and inconvenient'. The 1808 Act was promoted by Charles Watkin Williams Wynn (1775–1850), a forward thinking British politician who also rejoiced in the abolition of the slave trade. Due to his influence and endeavours, the 1808 Act unofficially became known as 'Mr Wynn's Act'.

Each county in England and Wales was obliged to build an asylum for their insane but fewer than twenty counties complied with the new Act. The remainder continued to rely on the old system of poor law, vagrancy law or criminal law. This left numerous pauper lunatics unprotected in institutions such as workhouses, gaols or indeed within their family homes where many were neglected.

In 1827 Lord Ashley, who became the 7th Earl of Shaftesbury on his father's death in 1851, became the Tory Member of Parliament for Woodstock, Oxfordshire and he, above many others, enacted profound and fundamental changes to the asylum system. Ashley served on the 1815 Select Committee on Pauper Lunatics in the House of Commons to determine the subject of lunacy and voted in favour of a motion the following year to amend the lunacy laws, the main defects of which were the lack of effective control over the admission, treatment and release of lunatics.

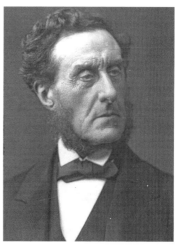

Earl of Shaftesbury, K.G. Photograph by John G. Murdoch. c. 1865.

A greater number of asylums were built in England and Wales following the subsequent 1828 *County Asylums (England) Act*, which increased the accountability of care for pauper lunatics. This Act was an important step forward in the fight against the wrongful incarceration of what some families termed 'inconvenient people' when the signatures of two doctors allowed for the easy removal of individuals under the previous lunacy Acts.

The Commission in Lunacy was established as a direct consequence of the 1828 Act, first for the Metropolis of London and then for the whole country. The Commissioners were a permanent body of inspectors made up of doctors and lawyers who had the power to prosecute unlawful practises and to prevent the renewal of licenses to madhouses and asylums not meeting required standards. The 1828 Act also made it a legal requirement for a medical superintendent to be provided at each asylum where the number of patients was greater than one hundred. At the same time the 1828 *Madhouses Act* was passed, repealing the previous *Madhouses Act* of 1774, making provision for the licensing and much needed regulation of such houses. Through these two Acts, fifteen commissioners were appointed for the Metropolis of London with Ashley being one of them.

Whilst, without doubt, these Acts moved things forward for the mentally ill, there remained five different auspices under which they could be held in 1832: private madhouses; the 1832 *County Asylum Act*; workhouses controlled by local authorities; Bethlehem (Bethlem) Royal

Hospital; and also as 'single' lunatics in private homes. Separate authorities administered these different forms of provision and there was no coordination between them; therefore, many individuals who were mentally ill were inadequately protected, both medically and legally, within the asylum and workhouse system.

By 1844, Ashley, having continually reviewed the conditions of asylums in the years following the 1828 *County Asylums Act*, motioned the House of Commons to consider an amended system of control and administration for the protection of confined lunatics. In an impassioned speech he stressed the importance of a system of control within asylums stating that:

> *it was the duty of the House to prescribe the conditions under which a man should be deprived of his liberty, and also those under which he might be released; it was their duty to take care that for those who required restraint, there should be provided kind and competent keepers, and that, while the patient received no injury, the public should be protected.*

Ashley commented upon the many horrors he had witnessed as a Lunacy Commissioner, and explained to the House that any man who had witnessed such cruelty to the 'most needy' of society would wish to help protect them. He pointed out that in many asylums there was a reluctance to help patients recover because the financial allowance for their care would then cease. As a result of the policy at that time, many patients were kept locked away with no hope of recovery or return to their families or communities.

Ashley's lobbying in the House of Commons brought about effective changes for the mentally ill in England and Wales. In 1845 after much discussion primarily concerning cost, a Lunacy Act and a County Asylums Act were given Royal assent within four days of each other. Both Acts were amendments to existing laws but strengthened the position under which patients in need of mental health provision should be cared for. One of the principal aims of the act was to ensure that every county and borough in England and Wales provided county asylum accommodation for all its pauper lunatics. It was believed that, in many cases, insanity was curable if it was treated early in an asylum. Due to the likely extensive costs that building an asylum would involve for each

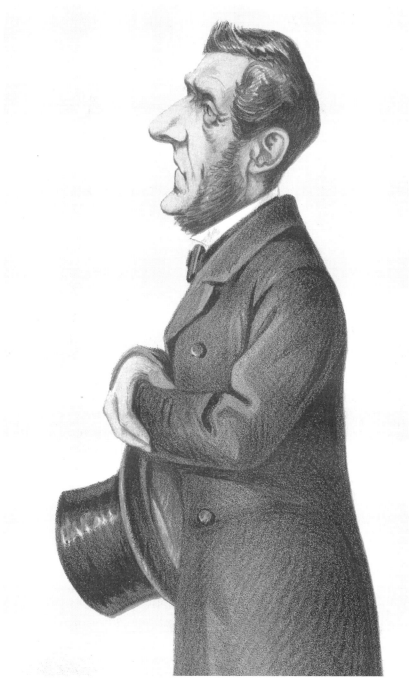

Earl of Shaftesbury. Caricature by Carlo Pellegrini. Vanity Fair, 1869.

county, many of the early objections were for financial reasons. These concerns were partly laid to rest by the opinion of Dr John Conolly (1794–1866), resident physician and alienist to the Middlesex County Asylum at Hanwell, who explained that many mentally ill people could be cured with appropriate early care. He believed that pauper lunatics were often housed in workhouses receiving no care due to a lack of appropriate facilities for their condition. Therefore, the construction of district asylums would eventually be a saving to communities, not an expense.

An article in *The Lancet* stated that the Acts 'will show that a provision is made for the treatment and preservation of all lunatics whose resources are inadequate ... and ... at the same time, every rational precaution is made to reduce, as far as possible the cost to the public'. Ashley described the Acts as 'a humane and economic way of dealing with pauper lunatics'.

There were other oppositions to the Acts. These came from a group of individuals who were concerned with the civil liberties of those likely to be affected by the changes to the law. One of these was John Thomas Perceval (1803–76), son of the former British prime minister Spencer Perceval who had been assassinated in 1809 in the lobby of the House of Commons by John Bellingham. Bellingham had been executed for the assassination as he claimed he had a grievance against the prime minister instead of pleading insanity at his trial.

John Thomas Perceval spent three years in a lunatic asylum in the 1830s. Placed there by his family, he spent the rest of his life highlighting the poor treatment he had received and in 1838 published a book entitled:

A narrative of the treatment experienced by a Gentleman during a state of mental derangement designed to explain the causes and nature of insanity, and to expose the injudicious conduct pursued towards many unfortunate sufferers under that calamity.

Under the terms of the 1845 *Lunacy Act*, a patient did not have the right to challenge their detention in an asylum but the 1845 *County Asylum Act* ensured that their county of origin had the responsibility to care for them. This caused concern that the government was becoming too powerful in the way they could determine the future of others without their knowledge or consent. However, when these two Acts gained Royal assent in August 1845, they became the basis of lunacy law until changes were made in 1890.

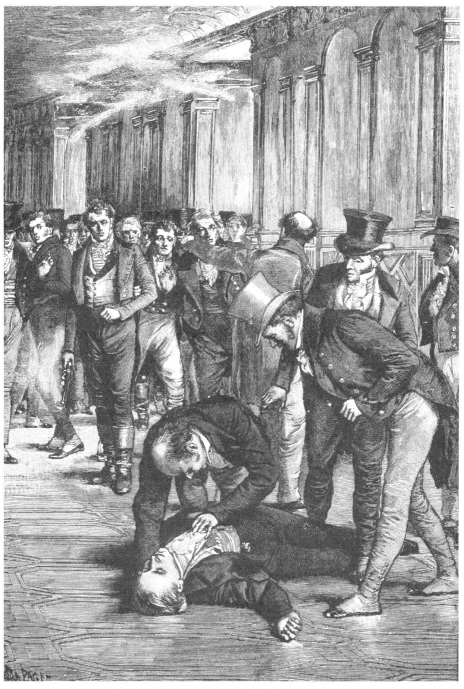

Assassination of Spencer Perceval. Cassell's Illustrated History of England, 1909.

Eleven Lunacy Commissioners were appointed as a result of the 1845 Lunacy Act to supervise the treatment of lunatics in England and Wales. Six commissioners (three medical and three legal) were employed full-time with a salary of £1,500 a year and the other five were honorary commissioners whose main function was to attend board meetings. They had national authority under the Lord Chancellor and Home Secretary over all asylums in England and Wales.

One of the main functions of the commissioners was to monitor the building of a network of publicly owned county asylums as required following the 1845 *County Asylums Act*. The Act also necessitated better record keeping in asylums and introduced stricter certification rules to protect individuals from wrongful incarceration. Two independent doctors were required to give statements stating their professional opinions as to why they considered a patient to be insane. From these more detailed records it is possible to draw a clearer profile of patients in terms of age, condition, family situation and social class, among other details. The Commissioners were responsible for the transfer of pauper lunatics from workhouses and other forms of outdoor relief to a public or private asylum, and regulated the treatment of patients in private asylums. They were obliged to visit asylums, private madhouses, hospitals, workhouses and gaols where there was at least one lunatic. Their findings were to be recorded in the visitors' book and a report made to the Commission noting any special circumstances.

This improvement to the regulations helped to shape the 'modern' nineteenth century asylum system which made staff accountable for the fair treatment of patients and individual counties obliged to provide adequate accommodation for their mentally ill. Asylums became the primary areas of care and society's response to mental health problems and medical superintendents formed the backbone of early psychiatry confining individuals often for many years as they attempted to understand and cure their illnesses.

As a Lunacy Commissioner, Ashley was against the use of restraint for the mentally ill and commended the pioneering work being carried out by the Tuke family at The Retreat in York and Dr John Conolly, resident physician and alienist to the Middlesex County Asylum at Hanwell.

Conolly became the focus of national attention following his appointment at Hanwell in 1839, as he removed all forms of mechanical

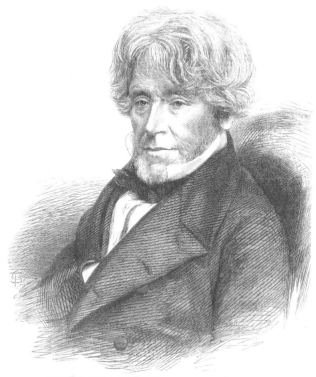

THE LATE DR. CONOLLY, RESIDENT PHYSICIAN OF HANWELL LUNATIC ASYLUM.

John Conolly, Resident Physician at Hanwell Lunatic Asylum.
Illustrated London News, 31 March 1866.

restraint for the patients and relied instead on moral therapy and kindly discipline. Initially, the new system of non-restraint was controversial. Many of Conolly's fellow alienists insisted that restraint was essential in the therapeutics of mental disorder. However, Ashley agreed with the methods of both Tuke and Conolly who, far from making lives easier for themselves by chaining up their patients and charging large fees, sought ways to help cure them of their insanity. Both The Retreat and Hanwell saw positive consequences for their patients by 1840.

In 1847, Conolly published *The Construction and Government of Lunatic Asylums*, which described the system and layout at Hanwell. It is clear that, despite not using measures of restraint, padded rooms were regularly used for patients' safety.

Patients in a very helpless state, or patients who have just had violent epileptic attacks, are often most securely placed in rooms in which there is a very low bedstead, and no other furniture, – or in rooms of which the whole floor is covered with bedding. Our padded rooms are much more frequently required for such patients than for violent patients, or for those disposed to strike their heads against the wall. Some of our paralytic patients, when reduced to a state of extreme helplessness, are placed in such rooms, and several of our epileptics, but when restraints were employed, such patients were fastened to common bedsteads, often in loose straw, and became violent from excess of physical misery. Restraint was the grand substitute for inspection, superintendence, cleanliness, and every kind attention. Troublesome patients were securely fastened down, and nobody seemed to care what condition they were in.

The same use of padded rooms also occurred at Parkside Asylum in Macclesfield, Cheshire in the latter half of the nineteenth century. Case notes from this asylum show that some patients chose to retreat to the padded rooms for comfort and solitude and that on these occasions the door was never locked.

On 15 January 1848, The *Illustrated London News* published details about non-restraint at Hanwell Asylum which was described as an 'experiment' but one that became used universally in the new asylums constructed following the 1845 Lunacy Act.

Seven years have elapsed since the experiment of non-restraint has been fully tried in the Hanwell Asylum; and Dr Conolly, in the spirit of a Christian philosopher, thanks God, with deep and unfeigned humility, that nothing has occurred during that period to throw discredit on the great principles for which he has so nobly battled.

In 1837, Dr William A.F. Browne (1805–85), when medical superintendent of the Montrose Royal Lunatic Asylum in Scotland, delivered a series of five seminal lectures to the managers of the asylum entitled '*What Asylums Were, Are, and Ought to be*'. They were published in one volume by Adam and Charles Black, Edinburgh, later that year. Dr

W.A.F. Browne became President of the Royal Medical Society, Edinburgh. He was an enthusiastic and practical leader and regarded education as part of his duties. In this work he highlighted the ideal asylum and outlined his philosophy for moral treatment of the insane within a secure and empathetic environment, rather than treatment by restraint, which had been very much the norm in the previous century. Browne may have adopted some of the philosophy of the Quakers at The Retreat in York, but he went much further and was more practical. Following publication of the lectures, Browne's ideas were widely followed by all asylums in Scotland.

Conceive a spacious building resembling the palace of a peer, airy, and elevated, and elegant, surrounded by extensive and swelling grounds and gardens. The sun and air are allowed to enter at every window, the view of the shrubberies and fields, and groups of labourers, is unobstructed by shutters or bars; all is clean, quiet and attractive. When you pass the lodge, it is as if you had entered the precincts of some vast emporium of manufacture; labour is divided, so that it may be easy and well performed, and so apportioned, that it may suit the tastes and powers of each labourer. You meet the gardener, the common agriculturist, the mower, the weeder, all intent on their several occupations, and loud in their merriment. The flowers are tended, and trained, and watered by one, the humbler task of preparing the vegetables for table is committed to another.

In line with this recommendation, and following the 1845 *Lunacy Act,* in 1856, the Commissioners in Lunacy issued official advice, suggestions and instructions in choosing sites for the construction and arrangement of new lunatic asylums. Although each asylum was individually designed, these guidelines were provided for the architects. It was recommended that the sites chosen for the buildings were large enough to accommodate agricultural and horticultural activities – not only for the employment of the patients but also for the daily management and provisioning of the asylum itself. There were recommendations that the main building should face south so that the patients' dayrooms and bedrooms had full benefit of the sun, which was likely to lift their mood. Their airing courts should also face south and be planted with trees and horticulturally landscaped.

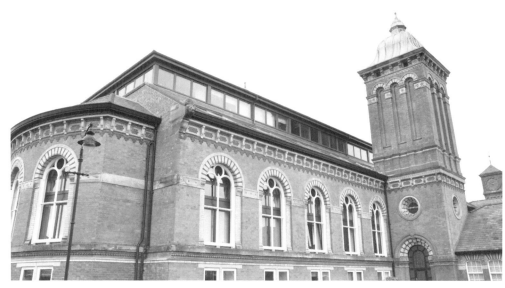

Parkside Asylum, water tower. © Kathryn Burtinshaw, 2015.

Access to the asylum should be kept to the north of the building so that the patients were not disturbed or overlooked by asylum visitors.

It was essential that each asylum had its own supply of fresh water and large water towers were built to accommodate this. The water towers became an iconic feature of the asylum, distinguishing the buildings that could otherwise be mistaken for palaces into places of refuge for the insane. As asylums were enlarged and improved some of the earliest additions were isolation wards, an infirmary and a place of worship.

Labouring work for the building of many of these asylums was carried out by the male patients. Work related activities were seen very much as beneficial for their therapeutic care. However, many historians have argued that this was exploitation and a low-cost way of procuring labour. During the construction of the new Cheshire Asylum in Macclesfield in the 1860s and 1870s, it was proposed by the asylum committee appointed to supervise the building that the first priority was the building of a male block so that '50 or 100 of the best patients could be transferred from Chester, who would do levelling, excavating and wheelbarrow work.'

By 1850 there were 7,140 patients living in twenty-four county and city asylums, and by 1860, only fifteen years after the 1845 Act, there were 15,845 patients resident in forty-one publicly funded county and city asylums. By 1910 this number had escalated to nearly 100,000 patients in ninety-one asylums across England and Wales. In 1880 it was estimated that ninety per cent of individuals in asylums were paupers funded at public expense and the remaining ten per cent were private patients funding their own care. From 1871, the decennial census of England and Wales included a disability column which specifically asked if individuals were 'deaf-and-dumb', 'blind', 'imbecile or idiot' or a 'lunatic'.

The income of those admitted to asylums varied, and from the middle of the nineteenth century many were admitted into institutionalised care as a result of reception orders made by medical practitioners and a justice of the peace. As reception orders took the form of a certificate, these individuals became known as 'certified' lunatics and their asylum care was funded by their union or parish. Described as pauper inmates in the records, not all of these people were specifically paupers, but they were in receipt of parish relief due to an inability to work because of their mental health disorder. Private asylum care was expensive and the fact that the majority of individuals were unable to afford it did not bar them from immediate treatment for their disorder. Many pauper lunatics admitted to asylums in the nineteenth century had occupations that would have enabled them to have a reasonable standard of living before insanity rendered them incapable of work.

It was widely acknowledged that individuals deemed to be insane were vulnerable from exploitation and for this reason, from as early as 1324, a statute entitled *De Prerogativa Regis* (By the King's Prerogative) was instituted to help protect them. This statute stated that the lands of lunatics 'shall be safely kept without Waste and Destruction, to be delivered unto them when they come to right mind'. During the nineteenth century this statute was strengthened, giving the Lord Chancellor powers to manage the estates of the insane. The *Lunacy Regulation Act* 1853 gave the courts power to sell or mortgage the estates of a lunatic to raise money to pay debts, and to enable his maintenance and stay within an asylum. Whilst in effect this appeared a harsh law, it was done to protect individuals who had valuable assets from being financially exploited from greedy creditors and family members. Because these cases were managed by the Lord Chancellor, those assessed were known as 'Chancery Lunatics'.

The *Criminal Lunatic Asylum Act* was passed in 1860 and was intended to provide a different level of asylum care and security for those individuals who had committed serious crimes but were found to be insane at the time of their offences. The subject of criminal insanity is examined in Chapter 12.

The *Lunacy Acts Amendment Act* of 1862 allowed Poor Law Unions to send chronic lunatics and imbeciles considered harmless and incurable into workhouse infirmary wards rather than to the pauper asylum. This was due to an escalation in overcrowding of the asylums and, in a report of the Poor Law Board, aimed '… to make more room for acute cases in which the treatment provided in the Lunatic Asylum is more important and necessary.' Although these workhouse wards had to comply with standards approved by the Lunacy Commission, using provision within workhouses was considerably cheaper than sending patients to asylums. Workhouses were deliberately harsh and unpleasant with inadequate food. For the poor insane who were less concerned about social stigmas, the new asylums of the nineteenth century were a much more comfortable alternative. One such patient was Sarah Ann Bennett, an epileptic who had been admitted to Macclesfield workhouse on ten occasions prior to her referral to an asylum in 1894. She expressed great gratitude for the move to the asylum, stating that the workhouse staff had mistreated her.

Following the creation of County Councils in 1888, further legislation to improve the asylum system was enacted in 1890 with a new *Lunacy Act*. This statute reviewed all aspects of the 1845 *Lunatic Asylums Act* and made changes and improvements to address the safety and comfort of patients admitted to mental health care in England and Wales after this period. One of the principal changes of the 1890 Act was the way in which patients should be processed when being admitted to the asylum system. Pauper patients no longer required an application from a relative – instead various authorities both medical and legal had a duty to bring individuals in need of asylum care before a magistrate, who asked for an opinion on their mental state from two doctors. This resulted in the issue of a 'Reception Order', which allowed for entry into an asylum. Reception Orders had to be renewed with the Lunacy Commissioners thereby proving that the patient was still in need of treatment within an asylum. These renewals were generally issued for one year, but longer requests for renewals were often made for individuals deemed to be incurable; five years was the longest period they could be issued for.

Other important changes were also made as a result of the 1890 legislation. Not only was the diet of patients considered but it also made provision for visits from friends and family. For the first time, asylums were required to keep an official record of those patients receiving restraint and the type of restraint and length of time it was used was recorded in a separate register. The continuation of recording patient details and medical treatment brought into force following the 1845 *Lunatic Asylums Act* remained as part of the new legislation of 1890.

The accountability of staff and the care of patients were at the forefront of the new Act and it remained the mainstay of legislation in England and Wales until its repeal with the *Mental Health Act* of 1959.

Legislation in Scotland

Under the *Act to Regulate Madhouses in Scotland* of 1815, 'every house kept for the reception of lunatics should be inspected at least two several [sic] times … in the year … by Sheriffs to be accompanied by such medical persons'. This Act allowed for fee-paying patients to be confined in institutions run by private individuals for profit. These establishments required annual licensing. Eight members from the Royal College of Physicians of Edinburgh and the Faculty of Physicians and Surgeons of Glasgow were elected as inspectors who sanctioned the renewal of licences. However, conditions in the madhouses were far from satisfactory.

Some legislation protected lunatics. *The Madhouses (Scotland) Act* of 1828 required houses containing 100 or more patients to have a resident physician or surgeon. Although this Act also required statutory registers of restraint to be kept, they seldom were, and restraint was used by attendants as an easy option, at their own discretion and without any records being made.

The Crichton Royal Institution for Lunatics at Dumfries was the last of seven prestigious, chartered asylums to be built, and it opened in 1839. Mrs Elizabeth Crichton, the institution's benefactor, invited Dr W.A.F. Browne to be its first medical superintendent. He moved from the Royal Lunatic Asylum at Montrose and held this post, and that of the resident physician, from its opening until 1857 when he was appointed a Commissioner of Lunacy.

In 1841, the *Madhouses, etc., (Scotland) Act* addressed 'dangerous lunatics' – defined as 'lunatics, who, if left to go at large, might be dangerous to the safety of the lieges.' Dangerous lunatics would be committed initially by the Procurator Fiscal to the local gaol or county prison as a place of safe custody until their condition was investigated by the Sheriff. If they were deemed to be insane, they would then be transferred to a lunatic asylum or private madhouse. They could be in prison for a number of weeks before transfer and were treated as ordinary criminals, deprived of all means of treatment, usually leaving in a worse mental condition than when they arrived. In some areas of Scotland, such as Edinburgh, the Procurator Fiscal could commit a dangerous lunatic directly to a chartered asylum.

'Criminal lunatics', defined under the *Prisons (Scotland) Act* of 1844, as being 'insane persons charged with serious offences', were committed to a special unit in the General Prison at Perth where they were treated as prisoners rather than patients. This massive and gloomy building was originally occupied by French prisoners of war from the Napoleonic wars, and was converted to a criminal lunatic establishment in October 1846. Inmates in other prisons throughout Scotland who became insane during their custodial sentence were also transferred to the Criminal Lunatic Unit at Perth Prison.

An Act for the Amendment and better Administration of the Laws relating to the Relief of the Poor in Scotland – known as the *Poor Law Amendment (Scotland) Act* of 1845 – removed the burden of providing poor relief from Church of Scotland parishes. This Act established parochial boards (later to evolve into Parish Councils and later into District Councils) to administer relief to the destitute and poor in the parishes throughout Scotland, and set up a central Board of Supervision for Relief of the Poor, based in Edinburgh. These parochial boards were authorised to raise taxes to fund poor relief through an assessed property rate. Following an application to the parochial board and an assessment by the parochial Inspector of Poor, some paupers qualified for 'outdoor relief' in the form of weekly assistance which could be money, food, clothing, shoes or coal. However, the majority of applicants were admitted to the 'poorhouse' – a building established to accommodate the destitute poor who could not work due to illness, inability or infirmity. The Poor Law Amendment (Scotland) Act required that every insane pauper should, within fourteen days of the onset of insanity, be taken to, and lodged in, an asylum or other place legally authorised to receive lunatics such as a licensed madhouse or poorhouse. It directed the inspectors of poor to report all cases of insanity chargeable in their respective parishes without delay to the Board of Supervision.

There were very few poorhouses before the 1845 Act. Those that did exist appear to have generally accepted insane and fatuous paupers without any sheriff's warrant. After the Act was passed, many new poorhouses were established. Parochial boards preferred to provide accommodation for their pauper lunatics in these establishments, as it was a cheaper option than sending them to public asylums or licensed madhouses. Separate wards for insane paupers were provided in a number of poorhouses, but elsewhere the insane mixed with the other inmates. There were local variations in the interpretation of the statutes as to which cases could be sent to a poorhouse. For example, in Aberdeenshire the sheriff ruled that only 'harmless' and 'incurable' lunatics could be admitted there, and only if accompanied by a medical certificate to confirm that there would be no hope of improvement of the patient's condition from treatment in an asylum. In the county of Fife, if a patient was quiet and manageable he would be sent to a poorhouse, but if 'refractory and violent' he would be admitted to an asylum where the cost of maintenance was higher. In other counties the rules were less stringent and all pauper lunatics, whether considered curable or not, could be admitted to a poorhouse that did not properly care for or supervise them, and had little intention or any means of curing them.

Poorhouses aimed to supply the insane with the most economical conditions, and to provide only the barest necessaries, to restore them to sanity. The cost of maintaining a pauper lunatic in the South Leith Poorhouse in 1855 was under £11 a year, which included provisions, clothing, staff salaries and rent. Patients slept in poorly furnished dormitories with limited, inadequate, and often soiled bedding. The poorhouses were generally overcrowded, badly ventilated and had inadequate heating and sanitary facilities. At the Dunfermline poorhouse 'tubs' were used in the dormitories rather than lavatories for the inmates and there were rooms for the seclusion of noisy cases. Personal restraint by means of straight-jackets and leather muffs was effected in most poorhouses at the discretion of attendants. Mortality rates for insane patients in poorhouses were considerably higher than in chartered asylums or licensed madhouses, with an early age at death. The average age at death for the Barony Poorhouse, Glasgow in 1854 was 39 years for males and 28 years for females.

One important proviso of the 1845 Poor Law (Scotland) Act was that the Board of Supervision was authorised to override the requirement to remove a patient to an asylum if it provided for his care and maintenance in some other manner. This resulted in a large number of single pauper lunatics being placed in the charge of relatives or unrelated keepers termed 'strangers'. This was particularly the case if the lunatic lived in remote counties some distance away from an asylum – thus in Caithness and Sutherland, over three-quarters of the insane poor were boarded out with relatives or strangers in 1855. The parochial medical officer was required to issue half-yearly certificates of insanity or fatuity, and confirm that the patient's condition was not likely to be aggravated by remaining in their current residence, but he was not required to state whether removal to an asylum would be beneficial to the patient. The cost to the parochial boards of boarding out a lunatic was less than half of the cost of maintenance in an asylum, and it also avoided the expense of transporting them there.

The costs of transporting a lunatic from a county that had no asylum to one that did were high. Patients from Orkney were sent to the Royal Asylum at Edinburgh, and those from Inverness, Caithness, Sutherland and Argyll to the asylums of Glasgow and Edinburgh, or to licensed madhouses in Midlothian. Undoubtedly, many pauper lunatics who should have been admitted to an asylum were boarded with relatives or strangers. Many were kept at home until they became violent or uncontrollable, and were harshly treated in their journey to the asylum, often manacled or physically restrained. Dr David Skae (1814–73), Resident Physician to Royal Edinburgh Asylum reported in 1855:

> *The cases from the northern counties are invariably incurable and hopeless before they reach me. They are generally cases of long standing. I believe this arises from unwillingness to increase the burdens on the parishes; there is a delay, on the part of inspectors of poor, in sending their patients. They are generally bound with canvas or with ropes on their arrival; and I have frequently seen ulcerations produced by the ropes. They are generally in a bad bodily condition.*
>
> *One of the patients was a soldier, who was paralytic and imbecile, yet his hands and feet were ironed, his hands being ironed behind his back. Another, who bore this painful and unnecessary treatment manfully during a long voyage from the North of Scotland, complained only of the disgrace of being led*

through the streets of Edinburgh in this humiliating state. He was to all appearance perfectly quiet and harmless, and has continued so since his admission.

Dorothea Dix (1802–87), a feminist social reformer, mental health agitator and philanthropist from New England, had already lobbied persistently to bring asylums to every American state when she visited Scotland on a moral crusade in 1855. She initially met resistance to her requests to visit Scottish asylums. When she did finally gain access to them she was alarmed by what she saw, and she made a number of successful representations to Queen Victoria and the British Parliament about the need to improve asylums in Scotland. Dorothea Dix was derided as an 'American Invader' and an 'interfering busybody', but she was instrumental in the instigation of the Royal Commission enquiry which started in 1855 and completed in 1857 'to inquire into the condition of lunatic asylums in Scotland, and the existing state of the law of that country in reference to lunatics and lunatic asylums'.

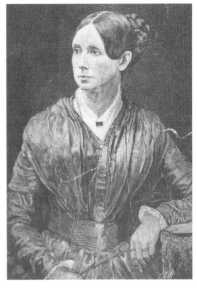

Dorothea L. Dix. Engraving by Richard Gordon Tietze.

The Royal Lunacy Commission for Scotland of 1855–7 reported on the grossly inadequate and appalling conditions in which many 'pauper lunatics' were incarcerated, under poor management and little regulation.

The chartered asylums, like the private licensed madhouses, were already overcrowded at that time. Although the chartered asylums were far superior to any other places where pauper lunatics could be admitted, there was a dearth of proper provision for these lunatics. The law required that pauper lunatics should be sent to public asylums, but failed to make any provision to build such establishments.

The Lunacy Commission report of 1857 gives some insights into how the asylums were run at that time from the reports of their inspections:

Dundee Royal Asylum was overcrowded and too many patients left under the charge of one attendant. The males and females are frequently placed two together in rooms originally attended for one patient. The airing courts for paupers are greatly overcrowded. There is deficiency in the means of personal cleanliness.

At Glasgow Royal Asylum the bedsteads of dirty patients have canvas bottoms and stand over troughs sunk in the floor which are flushed with water. This arrangement has a very offensive appearance, and it is calculated to degrade patients and encourage these faulty habits which it is intended to palliate.

In the Montrose Asylum dirty and destructive patients are permitted to be entirely naked while in seclusion, lying on the floor with no other bedding than loose straw and a blanket.

At Elgin Pauper Lunatic Asylum the single rooms were very imperfectly ventilated and not heated in any way. The bedsteads for wet patients have sloping bottoms with pipes leading into a tray or tub. There is no water-closet within doors. The patients are bathed once a week.

In several of the asylums, locks and straps are used to fasten the dresses of patients who would strip themselves.

At the Criminal Lunatic Wards of Perth Prison the whole arrangements are made with a view to the security of the patients without reference to their treatment as sufferers from disease. On 4th November 1856 we found three of the twenty-seven patients under restraint. One had an iron chain placed round his waist to which one hand was fastened; another had a hand fastened in a similar way and his legs were hobbled by rings placed round the ankles and connected together by an iron chain. The legs of the third were restrained in the same fashion.

The reports of inspections of the private institutions licensed for the reception of the insane (licensed madhouses), added as an appendix to the Royal Commission Report, were more alarming. There were a huge number of private madhouses in Musselburgh at that time:

At Hillend Asylum, Greenock, the bed-frames were dilapidated and saturated with filth; the quantity of straw in them was very scanty, and mixed with refuse; and that it was wet, offensive, soaked in urine, and broken into small portions, and had clearly not been renewed for a considerable time. That a certain number of patients, males as well as females, were stripped naked at night, and that in some cases two, or three, of them were placed to sleep in the same bed-frame, on loose straw, in a state of perfect nudity without any sheet. The patients are generally very dirty and untidy. Their feet were bare and very dirty, and their clothing ragged and filthy. Mechanical restraint is in habitual use. We noticed the attendant hiding a straight-waistcoat when we entered. A girl in the airing-ground had her arms manacled behind her back.

At Eastport House, Musselburgh one woman was in a straight-waistcoat and was described as very violent and destructive. She had broken her iron bedstead. In consequence of her violence she is often strapped to the bedstead. She was very poorly clad, scarcely with decency, and was in wretched condition. All the bedding in this room was very filthy.

At Lillybank House, Musselburgh there are no separate day-rooms, and the 72 patients are obliged to pass a great part of the day in their sleeping-rooms which are crowded with beds and generally contain no other furniture. The rooms have no means of ventilation and the atmosphere is extremely contaminated. The lower rooms are paved with bricks, impregnated with urine, and are constantly damp and offensive. There is no water on the premises; the supply for cooking and drinking is derived from a well in the street, and that for washing from the river. There are no water-closets in the house but there is a privy in each airing-ground, in which the excrement is allowed to accumulate till it forms a cartful for removal. The male patients presented unmistakable signs of deficient vital power. Their skins were cold, their circulation feeble, and their flesh wasted. They were poorly clothed without flannels and drawers, and were evidently underfed. Restraint is in common use with handcuffs, straps and straight-waistcoats. Some patients are chained to their beds at night.

At Whitehouse Asylum, Inveresk mechanical restraint is said to be seldom used – but we found one patient hand-cuffed as he is liable to sudden paroxysms of violent excitement preceding and following epileptic attacks.

After hearing and considering the evidence the Royal Commissioners published a damning report into the unsatisfactory provision for care of the insane in Scotland in 1857, particularly condemning the level of care awarded to pauper lunatics. They called for immediate action and *An Act for the Regulation of the Care and Treatment of Lunatics, and for the Provision, Maintenance, and Regulation of Lunatic Asylums in Scotland* – known as the 1857 *Lunacy (Scotland) Act* was passed on 25 August 1857. This Act made three major ground breaking changes. First, all insane patients had to be examined and certified by two doctors who were now required to give statements of facts or evidence to support their diagnosis of insanity; second, it created a General Board of Commissioners in Lunacy for Scotland to oversee the care of lunatics and to inspect and regulate asylums and licensed houses; and third, it divided Scotland into administrative Lunacy Districts each with a district board which were required 'to provide for the building of District Asylums for the reception of pauper lunatics and to ensure the proper care and treatment of lunatics generally, whether placed in asylums, or left in private houses under the care of relatives or strangers.' This was a paradigm shift from the haphazard local philanthropy behind the chartered asylums to formal central regulation backed by government funding.

Minor amendments were made to the 1857 Act by the 1862 *Lunacy (Scotland) Act* and the 1866 *Lunacy (Scotland) Act.* One provision of the 1862 Act was that public asylums were allowed to accept voluntary patients. However, the 1857 Act remained the principal lunacy legislation in Scotland until the twentieth century when the *Mental Deficiency and Lunacy (Scotland) Act* of 1913 increased state responsibility and changed the General Board of Commissioners in Lunacy for Scotland to the General Board of Control for Scotland, which allowed patients to admit themselves voluntarily to asylums.

Legislation in Ireland
At the beginning of the nineteenth century, the mentally ill in Ireland, who did not have families to care and support them, often became homeless and were left to wander the roads as destitute vagrants. This situation was due entirely to a complete lack of appropriate provision for their failing health needs. The 1804 House of Commons Select Committee Enquiry on the Aged and Infirm Poor of Ireland determined

that there was very sparse care available for 'idiots or insane persons'. In 1805, a *Bill for the Establishment of Provincial Asylums for Lunatics and Idiots in Ireland* was motioned by Sir John Newport, Member of Parliament for Waterford. This recommended the establishment of four provincial asylums, each of 250 beds, dedicated to the treatment of lunatics. Despite the enquiry, the Bill was opposed by party rivalry and some Members of Parliament were concerned about the costs and it would be a further ten years before the subject was raised and fully considered at government level again.

Throughout Ireland during the nineteenth century, there was a progressive increase in the number of people deemed to be insane. Despite the opening of new asylum provision at Grangegorman in Dublin in 1815, within two years there were grave concerns about the lack of beds for the mentally ill. This led to public and government concern about the rapid increase in the number of the mentally ill individuals, and anxiety about the already overstretched, inappropriate and inadequate facilities that were in place to deal with them. Following the Select Committee enquiries in England of 1815–16, Robert Peel, as Chief Secretary for Ireland and Chief Whip at Westminster (later to serve twice as Prime Minister of the United Kingdom from 1834–35 and 1841–46), initiated a Select Committee on the Lunatic Poor of Ireland to ascertain the provision for lunatics and idiots in every county. The Select Committee also attempted to assess the total number of insane persons and idiots under care in Ireland.

In 1817, aside from Dublin and County Cork, it was revealed that nineteen counties had no provision for their mentally ill and the remaining eleven counties declared a total of 989 idiots and insane in asylums, houses of industry, and gaols. Thomas Spring Rice (1790–1866), as governor of Limerick house of industry, made a tour of a number of houses of industry in southern Ireland and gave evidence to the enquiry. He reported on atrocious conditions in madhouses and called for reform of the treatment of the insane in Ireland. He optimistically believed that mental illness was transitory and could be cured if patients were given proper care and attention. Spring Rice described conditions as 'such as we should not appropriate for our dog-kennels'. He praised Dr William Hallaran's asylum at Cork, but severely criticised conditions at the Waterford and Clonmel Houses of Industry. Spring Rice wrote that conditions at Waterford resembled 'an ill-conducted gaol'. At Clonmel he found thirty-two lunatics – some of whom were lying naked on straw in a yard. Conditions at Limerick were even worse, with two patients having frozen to death.

> *In one of those rooms I found four and twenty individuals lying, some old, some infirm, one or two dying, some insane, and in the centre of the room was left a corpse of one who had died a few hours before. In the adjoining room I found a woman with the corpse of her child, lying upon her knees for two days; it was almost in a state of putridity. Furious persons were chained to their beds for years so that some lost the use of their limbs and were utterly incapable of moving.*

As a result of Spring Rice's report, the keeper at Limerick was dismissed and was replaced by male and female attendants loaned by Dr Hallaran of Cork. Hallaran's public asylum in Cork which, in 1792, was able to accommodate twenty-four patients, would later develop into the County and City of Cork Lunatic Asylum, accommodating 300 patients by 1822, and 500 by 1852. Further information on Irish asylums in the nineteenth century can be found at Chapter 7.

The Report of the Select Committee enquiry in Ireland of 1817 found that twenty-three of the thirty-two counties of Ireland made absolutely no provision for lunatics although the grand juries had power to provide funds for this purpose under a 1787 act of the Irish Parliament. It supported the establishment of a system of asylums. Their reasons were twofold: it gave the possibility of effective treatment for lunatics; and, by removing the insane from overcrowded infirmaries, gaols and workhouses, these places would operate more efficiently and effectively.

Spring Rice entered parliament as Member for Limerick in 1820 and was instrumental in encouraging speedy implementation of legislation for asylum reform. Subsequently the *Lunacy (Ireland) Act* of 1821 was passed giving the Lord Lieutenant (the chief administrator of the British Government in Ireland, based at Dublin Castle) the much needed powers to establish asylums for the lunatic poor throughout Ireland. The new asylums were funded both by central government at national level, and by grand juries locally. The establishment, regulation and planning of asylums was controlled centrally by Commissioners for General Control and Correspondence. Each asylum had its own Board of Governors who met monthly with local responsibility to direct asylum activities. Members were typically landed gentry, magistrates, merchants, traders, and clergymen. The Irish asylum system differed from other parts of the United Kingdom in that it operated independently of the Poor Law. Both paying patients and paupers could be admitted to the publically funded district asylums. The 1821 Act also provided that criminal lunatics would be detained in these asylums at the pleasure of the Lord Lieutenant. This was different from the practise in England and Wales where they could be detained in gaols.

Under the 1826 *Prisons (Ireland) Act*, private asylums had to be inspected by the Inspector-General of Prisons. This changed in 1842 with the *Private Lunatic Asylums (Ireland) Act* which required private asylums to be licensed on an annual basis and to be visited by the inspectors of lunatics. Patients could only be detained in a private asylum on an order made out by a relative or friend accompanied by the certificates of two medical practitioners who had separately examined the patient.

The 1838 *Criminal Lunatics (Ireland) Act*, often referred to as the *'Dangerous Lunatics Act'*, provided a separate form of admission when an individual was arrested under circumstances suggesting that they were of deranged mind and were dangerous. Such alleged lunatics could be detained indefinitely by two justices of the peace, acting on a sworn statement by a third party – usually a relative. The justices were empowered, but not required, to seek the opinion of a medical practitioner to examine the suspect and to inform their decision. The justices could commit a 'dangerous lunatic' initially to a gaol. The person would remain in gaol until discharged by an order of two justices or until transferred to a district asylum by warrant of the Lord Lieutenant when a place became available. Such lunatics admitted to asylums could only be discharged when two doctors certified that they had 'become of sound mind' and by an order of the Lord Lieutenant.

In 1843, new Privy Council Rules were introduced by the Lord Lieutenant for all district asylums in Ireland, restricting the powers of the lay manager and increasing those of the visiting physician. These rules also allowed for the provision of religious services and permitted clergymen to visit patients at the patient's request. The Privy Council Rules stipulated that both Roman Catholic and Church of Ireland chaplains and chapels should be provided in all Irish asylums. Asylum physicians could veto patients suffering from 'excessive religious enthusiasm, mania or excitement' from attending any service.

The 1846 *Lunatic Asylums (Ireland) Act* removed the necessity of an order of the Lord Lieutenant to discharge a recovered lunatic. Unfortunately, the 'dangerous lunacy' procedures made the committal of lunatics relatively easy in Ireland and were commonly subject to abuse and misuse. Many sick patients, who were not at all dangerous, were committed under this legislation. They were automatically criminalised as they had 'threatened violence' towards others. Many patients spent weeks or months in gaol before being transferred to an asylum. The report of the inspectors of lunatics in 1847 noted that forty per cent of committals had been in gaol for over a year.

The 1845 *Central Criminal Lunatic Asylum (Ireland) Act* directed that there should be only 'one central asylum for insane persons charged with offences in Ireland, in or near the City of Dublin' to provide psychiatric treatment for individuals who were insane at the time a crime was committed, or at the time of indictment and were acquitted on grounds of insanity but detained 'at the pleasure of the Lord Lieutenant'. Subsequently, Dundrum Asylum for the Criminal Insane was opened in 1850 on the outskirts of Dublin. It was considered to be the first secure hospital in Europe, predating Broadmoor in England. It did not take every criminal lunatic, but only those who had committed heinous crimes such as murder and were found guilty but insane. This Act also provided that someone who had been committed as a 'dangerous' lunatic could be considered for discharge if they had ceased to be dangerous. The Act also established the Inspectorate of Lunacy. The first two Inspectors of Lunacy in Ireland were Dr Francis White and Sir John Nugent who were appointed in 1846 and 1847 respectively. Chapter 12 contains additional information on 'The Criminal Lunatic'.

The 'dangerous lunatic' procedures of the 1838 Act were exploited and used inappropriately on a regular basis. In 1847 the Inspectors of Lunacy reported that almost half of committals under the Act were made without a medical opinion. There was no mandatory review of the condition and status of someone detained under the *Dangerous Lunatics Act*. The proportion of 'dangerous' as opposed to 'ordinary' lunatics increased as the century progressed and the asylums became overcrowded. In 1865 there were over 500 'dangerous lunatics' in gaols awaiting transfer to asylums; prison governors were unhappy that the presence of lunatics disrupted prison discipline. Asylum doctors believed that the earlier a lunatic was admitted to an asylum, the greater their chance of cure. Subsequently, amendments were made under the 1867 *Lunacy (Ireland) Act* whereby suspected 'dangerous' lunatics were committed by two justices directly to an asylum rather than a gaol for assessment, and it became mandatory to obtain a medical certificate from the medical officer of the dispensary district in which they were sitting. Dispensary doctors were salaried officers of the Irish poor law medical system set up in 1853.

The Inspectors of Lunacy advised magistrates that they should only use their powers under the 1867 Act against people likely to be violent or commit a crime. The asylums could not legally refuse to admit a patient under the Act, even when the asylum staff felt the patient was better suited to a workhouse environment, or was not actually insane. There remained a high proportion of admissions to district lunatic asylums classified as 'dangerous' throughout the latter part of the nineteenth century – seventy-six per cent of male admissions and sixty-seven per cent of female admissions to Irish asylums in the period 1890-92 were labelled as 'dangerous lunatics'.

The 1875 *Lunatic Asylums (Ireland) Act* allowed for the transfer of any chronic lunatic who was not dangerous, from the asylum to the workhouse on a certificate from the resident medical superintendent as fit and proper to be removed. It also empowered asylum managers to retake an escaped lunatic without new certificates within fourteen days of the escape.

The 1875 *Lunatic Asylums (Ireland) Act* remained in force until the end of the nineteenth century and some minor amendments were made in 1901 by the *Lunacy (Ireland) Act: An Act to amend the Law relating to Lunatics in Ireland.* The 1883 *Trial of Lunatics (Ireland) Act* allowed a jury to return a verdict of 'guilty but insane' for a person found to be insane at the time of any indictable offence including murder.

The *Local Government (Ireland) Act* of 1898 established County and District Councils in Ireland and shifted the responsibility of 'providing and maintaining sufficient accommodation for the lunatic poor in accordance with the Lunatic Asylums Acts' away from central control by Boards of Guardians and Grand Juries onto the individual county councils.

Despite several government commissions into the conditions of overcrowding in asylums in Ireland, it was not until the *Mental Treatment Act* of 1945 that there was an overall process of reform.

Chapter 4

English Asylums in the
Nineteenth Century

The *County Asylums Act* or 'Wynn's Act' of 1808, made it an obligation for counties to build asylums for those who were judged to be insane (see Chapter 3). These were not intended as curative establishments, but places to detain the mentally ill away from the rest of society. As a result, several counties began to make arrangements to build new accommodation for their insane. However, by the time of the 1815 Select Committee Enquiry on the Better Regulation of Madhouses very few county asylums were actually operational in England. The first was the General Lunatic Asylum at Nottingham.

The committee praised the standard of care and treatment at this asylum, which had been jointly funded by the county ratepayers and by voluntary subscriptions. Following Wynn's Act, Nottinghamshire had determined that it had fifty-six lunatics in the county, and built its new asylum to house eighty patients. The new asylum at Sneinton in Nottinghamshire, modelled both in terms of architecture and treatment on The Retreat at York, opened its doors to patients in 1812; the county soon discovered that the number of patients requiring care exceeded the availability of beds. Within the next eighty years, the asylum at Sneinton had expanded and obtained additional premises as the need for accommodation escalated.

The second county asylum to open was at Bedford; the mastermind of Samuel Whitbread (1764–1815), son of the brewer Samuel Whitbread (1720–96). Whitbread was Member of Parliament for Bedford from 1790 to 1813 and a keen supporter of civil and religious rights. He was a great admirer of Napoleon and sank into a depression following his abdication in 1814. Whitbread committed suicide by cutting his throat with a razor the following year. The asylum at Bedford fell short of expectations due to huge overcrowding and a lack of staff. As the neighbouring counties of Hertfordshire and Huntingdonshire had failed to build their own asylums, they sent their insane to Bedford. Consequently, there was a patient population explosion, which led to the building of The Stotfold Three Counties Asylum in Hitchin, Hertfordshire. Opened in March 1860, by 1861 it accommodated 460 patients.

In 1809, magistrates in Norfolk appointed a committee to determine the number of lunatics and insane persons within the county. It concluded that, as there were 153, a county asylum was needed and the Norfolk County Asylum opened in Norwich in 1814. The buildings were originally designed to accommodate about 100 patients and in the early years there were about seventy patients housed in the asylum. Later extensions in 1831 and 1840 allowed this number to double and more substantial additions in the late 1850s, and the construction of an additional asylum building completed in 1881, provided care for 700 inpatients.

The first pauper lunatic asylum for the county of Middlesex opened in June 1831 at Hanwell; at that time, Middlesex encompassed many areas that would be considered part of London today. Originally built to accommodate 500 patients, an increasing demand for asylum provision required the building to be extended in 1831, 1837, 1857 and 1879. Hanwell became prominent in the field of early psychiatry due to the work of two of its first medical superintendents. Dr (later Sir) William Ellis (1780–1839) was the first of those, in charge of Hanwell between 1831 and 1833. Ellis had previously been medical superintendent at the West Riding Pauper Asylum in Wakefield, West Yorkshire from the time of its instigation in 1818. He and his wife Mildred, who acted as the asylum Matron, had impressed with their moral and religious convictions and their wish to ensure that patients recovered their self-esteem. Ellis introduced his idea of 'Therapy of Employment', which encouraged patients to use the skills and trades they had acquired before entering the asylum, not only to occupy themselves and aid in their treatment by restoring their self-respect, but also for the benefit of the asylum. Some historians believe, perhaps correctly, that this system was abused in many asylums, but a writer of the time, having visited Hanwell, recorded her thoughts on a system she believed to be of benefit to the patients.

Tait's *Edinburgh Magazine* published an account of a visit by Miss Harriet Martineau (1802–76) to Hanwell in June 1834. Harriet Martineau was born in Norwich into an upper-middle class family who fell into financial difficulties in the late 1820s. Harriet began to make a name for herself as a writer and made comparative studies on social institutions, one of which was Hanwell Asylum.

It is commonly agreed that the most deplorable spectacle which society presents, is that of a receptacle for the insane. In pauper asylums we see chains and strait-waistcoats, – three or four half-naked creatures thrust into a chamber filled with straw, to exasperate each other with their clamour and attempts at violence; or else gibbering in idleness, or moping in solitude. In private asylums, where the rich patients are supposed to be well taken care of in proportion to the quantity of money expended on their account, there is as much idleness, moping, raving, exasperating infliction, and destitution of sympathy, though the horror is attempted to be veiled by a more decent arrangement of externals. Must these things be?

I have lately been backwards and forwards at the Hanwell Asylum for the reception of the pauper lunatics of the county of Middlesex. On entering the gate, I met a patient going to his garden work with his tools in his hand, and passed three others breaking clods with their forks, and keeping near each other for the sake of being sociable. Further on, were three women rolling the grass in company; one of whom, – a merry creature, who clapped her hands at the sight of visitors, had been chained to her bed for seven years before she was brought hither, but is likely to give little further trouble, henceforth, than that of finding her enough to do. A very little suffices for the happiness of one on whom seven years of gratuitous misery have been inflicted; – a promise from Mrs Ellis to shake hands with her when she has washed her hands, – a summons to assist in carrying in dinner, – a permission to help to beautify the garden, are enough. Further on, is another in a quieter state of content, always calling to mind the strawberries and cream Mrs Ellis set before the inmates on the lawn last year, and persuading herself that the strawberries could not grow, nor the garden get on without her, and fiddle-faddling in the sunshine to her own satisfaction and that of her guardians. This woman had been in a strait-waistcoat for ten years before she was sent to Hanwell. In a shed in this garden, sit three or four patients cutting potatoes for seed, singing and amusing each other; while Thomas, – a mild, contented looking patient, passes by with Mrs Ellis's clogs, which he stoops to tie on with all possible politeness; finding it much pleasanter, as Dr Ellis says, 'to wait on a lady than be chained in a cell'.

Dr John Conolly (1794–1866), the third medical superintendent at Hanwell and its visiting physician between 1839 and 1852, abolished the use of mechanical restraints to control patients at the asylum and as such, Hanwell became the model on which many other asylums went on to treat their patients. In 1852, Conolly became the local physician and supervised the opening of the County Lunatic Asylum at Hatton Park in Warwickshire. The first patients to arrive were treated under his regime of moral therapy. Conolly very much adopted the practice of the Tuke family at The Retreat at York and that of Robert Gardiner Hill (1811–78) at Lincoln. Far less well known than John Conolly, Robert Gardiner Hill was appointed medical superintendent of the Lincoln Lunatic Asylum in 1835 where he was possibly the first to run a pauper asylum without the use of mechanical restraint. In 1857 he published a book entitled *A Concise History of the Entire Abolition of Mechanical Restraint in the Treatment of the Insane.* The following extract from his book sums up his thoughts on the subject.

Classification and watchfulness. Vigilant and unceasing attendance by day and by night. Kindness, occupation and attention to health, cleanliness and comfort; and the total absence of every description of other occupation of the Attendants. This treatment in a properly constructed and suitable building, with a sufficient number of strong and active attendants always at their post, is best calculated to restore the patient; and all instruments of coercion and torture are rendered absolutely and in every case unnecessary.

Another early alienist with forward thinking views about the treatment of patients in asylums was Thomas Octavius Prichard (1808–47). Prichard had been the medical superintendent at Glasgow Royal Lunatic Asylum before being appointed as medical superintendent at the newly opened Northamptonshire County General Lunatic Asylum in 1838. He was also an early advocate of 'moral management', the humane treatment of the mentally ill. When the poet John Clare (1793–1864) entered Northamptonshire Asylum in 1841, Prichard encouraged him to continue his writing and one of his most famous poems, *I Am,* was written while he was a patient there. Clare died in the asylum in 1864.

Whilst Hanwell was one of the earliest pauper asylums to open following the 1828 *County Asylums (England) Act*, two other counties had already established care for their pauper insane. Cheshire County Lunatic Asylum, in Chester, which later became known as The Deva Asylum, opened in 1829. It was intended to provide for the care and maintenance of pauper and criminal lunatics. Originally designed to accommodate ninety patients, it was staffed by a matron and twelve attendants but did not have a resident medical superintendent until the early 1850s, at which point the patient population had increased to over 200. Some of the earliest patients at Chester were Welsh lunatics with little command of the English language. This was due to Chester's proximity to the Welsh border counties of Denbighshire and Flintshire, and the lack of asylum care in North Wales until the mid-1840s. These patients returned to Wales following the construction of the asylum at Denbigh in 1848.

Despite the removal of Welsh lunatics, the asylum at Chester continued to expand. By 1871, the patient population had increased to 553, and was staffed by a medical superintendent, an assistant medical officer, a matron and over fifty attendants.

Cheshire had anticipated the need for additional asylum provision in the county from the mid-1860s following recommendations by Dr Thomas Nadauld Brushfield (1828–1910) who graduated as a Doctor of Medicine from the University of St Andrews in 1862 and was the medical superintendent of the asylum at Chester. Recommendations were made to the Court of Quarter Sessions by the visiting justices of the asylum in 1865 that further accommodation should be provided within the county due to the increased number of pauper lunatics. As a result, it was decided that a second facility for the pauper insane of Cheshire should be built at Macclesfield. This second asylum, Parkside, was opened in 1871 having been partly constructed using the workforce of the male patients at Chester to excavate and level the ground.

As the numbers of insane grew, England witnessed an explosion in the provision of institutions to care for them. Few English counties had only one asylum by the end of the nineteenth century and many counties had multiple establishments catering for a wide range of different needs. By 1851, the first county lunatic asylum in Lancashire, built in Lancaster in 1816, could no longer cope with the large numbers of pauper lunatics that

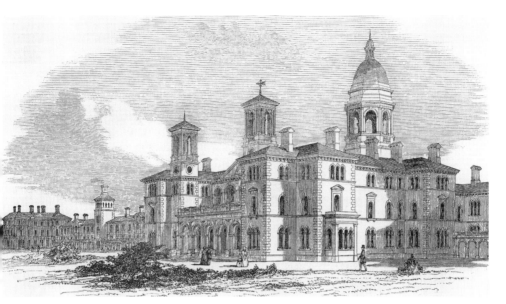

Middlesex Pauper Lunatic Asylum, Colney Hatch. Illustrated London News, 1849.

the progress of industrialisation, and the expansion of both Liverpool and Manchester as cities of commerce, inevitably produced. This led to an increased need in care for the county's insane and so two new asylums were built at Rainhill and Prestwich respectively.

Despite the extra provision in Lancashire, by 1866, the asylums at Lancaster, Rainhill and Prestwich were full and a fourth asylum at Whittingham near Preston was built. As in Cheshire, male patients from the other asylums helped with the construction work and Whittingham formally opened in 1873 with beds for 1,000 patients.

Middlesex also expanded its provision for the insane in 1851 with the construction of a second asylum in North London. Known as the Second Middlesex County Asylum or Colney Hatch Lunatic Asylum, it had the capacity to treat 1,000 patients and catered predominantly for those living in north and east London. Before it was built, Dr John Conolly wrote a long letter to Benjamin Rotch (1794–1854), Chairman of the Committee of Visitors, expressing his expertise in the construction of asylums for the comfort of the patients. Not only did he stress the need to prevent the use of mechanical restraint, but he also warned about potential fire hazards and recommended that all parts of the asylum including the staircases should be constructed of brick or stone. Rotch, who was also Member of Parliament for Knaresborough, was influential in decisions on asylum design due to his position both in parliament and within the Lunacy Commission.

Colney Hatch was huge – at the time of its construction it was the largest asylum in Britain with six miles of corridors including the longest corridor in Britain. There were two medical superintendents, one for male patients and another for females. Due to its location and catchment area, it contained a large number of Jewish patients, inhabitants of the East End of London. To cater for the needs of this group of people, the asylum installed a kosher kitchen and employed a Yiddish-speaking attendant to assist with communication. A church and burial ground were consecrated by the Bishop of London when it opened in 1851 but, by 1873, the burial ground was disused and a memorial marking its place recorded that:

In this consecrated ground
Have been interred
the remains of
2,696 inmates of this asylum,
and this monument
has been erected
to their memory
by the Committee of Visitors
January 1883

Despite its immense size, it rapidly became too small to accommodate the swelling numbers of patients who needed asylum care. Despite expansion throughout the 1850s so that patient numbers could be increased to 2,000, by 1867, 3,800 applications had been turned down due to the shortage of beds. Many of the new structures constructed to accommodate additional patients were built of wood and a fire at the asylum in January 1903 quickly took hold in a Jewish dormitory killing fifty-one female patients. Lack of space at Colney Hatch meant it was inevitable that Middlesex needed a third county asylum. Banstead Asylum in Banstead, Surrey fulfilled this role when it opened in 1877.

Many patients waited in desperate circumstances in workhouses ill-equipped to deal with them until an asylum place could be found. Poor Law doctors, although not alienists, quickly became accustomed to dealing with insane inmates – a situation that Poor Law officials were keen to maintain as it was a lot cheaper to house an individual in a workhouse than in one of the new county asylums. Some pauper patients wished to be transferred to an asylum as the living conditions, food, and overall level of care, was superior. The new asylums resembled palaces, with theatres, tennis courts and ballrooms and were a far cry from the austere surroundings of the local workhouse.

Case study: Sarah Ann Bennett

Sarah Ann Bennett had been admitted and discharged from Macclesfield workhouse on ten occasions before being transferred to Parkside Asylum on 24 April 1894 due to epileptic seizures. She said that the attendants at the workhouse had ill-treated her and that she was always put into a padded room when she was having seizures. Her asylum case notes reveal that she seemed very satisfied to be in the asylum. Mary Ann Bolton also expressed the same opinion of her transfer from Nottingham workhouse to Parkside in 1884. Mary Ann suffered from acute mania and hallucinations but she expressed a horror at being returned to the workhouse and stated that she was very comfortable in the asylum.

The satisfaction of former workhouse patients with the surroundings of Parkside is understandable. The building was constructed using local but high quality materials. It was warm, due to heating provided by hot water pipes, and well vented to prevent the spread of infectious diseases. Internal bathrooms with hot and cold running water and water closets were installed, complete with mahogany fixtures and fittings. The main hall, which was used for dances and balls, had a dance floor made of maple and was considered to be the best in the north of England. Food was adequate and of reasonable quality. The nurses and attendants wore ordinary dress and patients were permitted to wear their own clothes. For those who had insufficient apparel, clothing was issued in the form of wool or cotton dresses and plaid shawls.

Undoubtedly the influence of men such as Lord Shaftesbury had a profound influence in the move towards improved conditions for the insane in the nineteenth century. Similarly an increasing number of medical men were making breakthroughs in the early psychiatric treatment of mental health disorders. However, in many cases it was finance that prevented some asylums from being built quickly. Shaftesbury was a brilliant orator, but when he made a public appeal at the London Freemasons' Hall in 1861 for donations towards the establishment of a 'Benevolent Asylum for the Insane of the Middle Classes', he was unaware of the effect this had on Thomas Holloway.

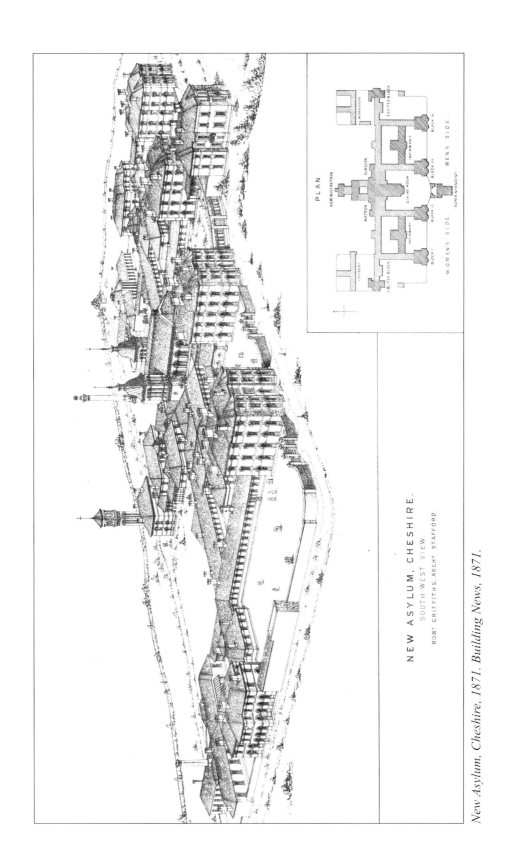

New Asylum, Cheshire, 1871. Building News, 1871.

Holloway was a multi-millionaire philanthropist who had made his money from the sale of patent medicines designed to cure all illnesses. He made the decision to give part of his fortune as a charitable donation and therefore determined to provide a place of refuge for the temporarily deranged middle classes so that they could be assisted to resume their working lives. As a result, he paid for Holloway Sanatorium at Virginia Water in Surrey. The enterprise cost more that £300,000 when it opened in 1885. The sanatorium was run along similar lines to an English country house with elegant rooms and furniture and manicured grounds. There was a stronger emphasis on recreation rather than employment as in pauper asylums because the class of patient residing at Holloway was not used to many forms of manual work. The fees were dependent on individual circumstances, with better-off patients paying more to subsidise the cost to the equally deserving but less affluent. The Holloway Sanatorium was very much conceived along the lines of social class. The middle classes were often unable to pay the fees of private asylums but were reluctant to access county pauper asylums due to social stigma and the perceived detriment to their recovery. Holloway bridged the gap between the two, but was very much a unique institution. The first available census for the sanatorium in 1891 reveals that the patients originated from a substantial distance to the establishment and comprised a variety of occupations including Royal Naval officers, clerks at the London Stock Exchange and many individuals living on their own means.

Private asylums or madhouses had existed in England for many centuries and some remained in the nineteenth century for the more elite clientele, charging large fees. One such asylum, Ticehurst House in Sussex, opened in 1792 – pre-dating The York Retreat by four years. Ticehurst, like the Bethlehem hospital in London, was run by four successive generations of the same family, the Newingtons, until 1917. Ticehurst developed into a grandiose estate covering about 500 acres, part of which was landscaped to mimic Kew Gardens. Its facilities attracted a higher class of patient and standards of care were based on empathy, benevolence and sanctuary. It became so desirable in terms of psychiatric care that it was able to choose its patients.

Nevertheless, county pauper asylums formed the backbone of mental health care in England during the nineteenth century. As patient numbers increased so did the need for extra beds. What had started at the beginning of the nineteenth century as optimistic assistance for those in need of mental help, soon spiralled out of control as the newly built asylums became overcrowded.

The following is a list of asylums built in England during the nineteenth century. These asylums were predominantly built for the pauper insane.

Year	Name and location of establishment
1811	*The General Lunatic Asylum*, Nottingham also known as *Sneinton Asylum.*
1812	*Bedford Lunatic Asylum*, Bedford, Bedfordshire.
1814	*Norfolk County Asylum,* also known as *St Andrew's Hospital*, Norwich.
1815	*Cornwall County Lunatic Asylum*, Bodmin, Cornwall.
1816	*Lancaster County Lunatic Asylum* also known as *Lancaster Moor Hospital*, Lancaster. This was Lancashire's first county lunatic asylum.
1818	*Stafford County Lunatic Asylum*, also known as *St George's Hospital*, Stafford.
1818	*West Riding County Asylum*, Wakefield, Yorkshire. This was the first asylum for the West Riding of Yorkshire.
1819	*Lincoln Lunatic Asylum*. This was renamed *The Lawn Hospital for the Insane* in 1885.
1823	*Gloucestershire First County Asylum* in Gloucester.
1826	*Oxford Lunatic Asylum*, Headington, Oxfordshire. Later known as the *Radcliffe Lunatic Asylum* and then the *Warneford Lunatic Asylum*.
1829	*Cheshire County Lunatic Asylum*, Chester. Later known as *The Deva Asylum*.
1829	*Suffolk County Asylum for Pauper Lunatics*, Melton, Suffolk.
1831	*Middlesex County Asylum* at Hanwell. Later known as *London County Asylum*, Hanwell.
1832	*Dorset County Asylum* at Forston House in Charminster.
1833	*Kent County Asylum* in Barming Heath near Maidstone. Later known as *Oakwood Hospital*.
1837	*Leicestershire County Asylum*. Later known as *Leicestershire and Rutland Lunatic Asylum*.
1838	*Northampton General Lunatic Asylum*. The name was changed to *Northampton General Lunatic Asylum for the Middle and*

	Upper Classes in 1876 when a separate County Lunatic Asylum for pauper patients was opened in Upton, Northampton. It was renamed *St Andrew's Hospital for Mental Diseases* in 1887.
1841	*Surrey County Asylum* in Springfield Park in Wandsworth.
1845	*Devon County Pauper Lunatic Asylum* in Exeter at Exminster.
1845	*New Shropshire Lunatic Asylum* in Bicton Heath. Later known as *The Lunatic Asylum for the Counties of Salop and Montgomery, and for the Borough of Wenlock* and *The Lunatic Asylum, for the Counties of Salop and Montgomery, and for the Borough of Much Wenlock*.
1846	*Oxford County Pauper Lunatic Asylum* in Littlemore, Oxford. Later known as *Littlemore Asylum*.
1847	*The Asylum for Idiots in Park House*, Highgate, London. Relocated to Redhill, Surrey in 1855 and was renamed *The Earlswood Asylum For Idiots* but was also known as *The Royal Earlswood Hospital*.
1847	*North and East Ridings Asylum*, York. Later known as *Clifton Asylum*.
1848	*Somerset And Bath County Asylum at Wells*, Somerset. Later known as The *Mendip Hospital, Wells and Somerset and Bath Pauper Lunatic Asylum*.
1849	*Hull Borough Lunatic Asylum* formerly the *Hull and East Riding Refuge*.
1849	*Wiltshire County Asylum* at Devizes, Wiltshire. Later known as *Roundway Hospital*.
1850	*Birmingham Borough Asylum*. Later known as *All Saints Mental Asylum* and *Winson Green Asylum*.
1851	*Derby County Asylum* in Mickleover, Derbyshire. Later known as *Derby County Mental Hospital* and *The Pastures Hospital*.
1851	*Middlesex County Pauper Asylum*, also known as *Colney Hatch Lunatic Asylum* in north London and *Friern Hospital*. This was the second county asylum for Middlesex.
1851	*Prestwich Asylum* in Prestwich, Manchester. This was a second county asylum for Lancashire.
1851	*Lancashire County Asylum* known as *County Lunatic Asylum, Rainhill* from about 1861. Located at Rainhill, Liverpool. This was the third county asylum for Lancashire.
1852	*Hampshire County Lunatic Asylum* in Fareham, Hampshire. Later known as *Knowle Mental Hospital*.

1852	*Lincolnshire County Lunatic Asylum* also known as *Lindsey, Holland, Lincoln and Grimsby District Pauper Lunatic Asylum* and *Bracebridge Pauper Lunatic Asylum*. Situated in Bracebridge, Lincolnshire.
1852	*Warwick County Lunatic Asylum* in Hatton, Warwickshire. Later known as *Hatton County Lunatic Asylum*.
1852	*Worcester County Pauper and Lunatic Asylum* in Powick, Worcestershire. Later known as *Powick Lunatic Asylum*.
1853	*Buckinghamshire County Lunatic Asylum* in Stone, Buckinghamshire.
1853	*Essex County Lunatic Asylum* in Brentwood, Essex. Later known as *Brentwood Mental Hospital*.
1855	*The Earlswood Asylum For Idiots* in Redhill, Surrey also known as *The Royal Earlswood Hospital*. Known as the *Asylum for Idiots* when it opened in 1847 in Park House, Highgate, London.
1858	*Isle of Ely and Borough of Cambridge Pauper Lunatic Asylum* in Cambridge. Later known as *Cambridgeshire County Asylum*, then *Fulbourn Hospital*.
1859	*Asylum for Lunatic Paupers of Durham* in Durham. Later known as *Sedgefield Lunatic Asylum*.
1859	*County Pauper Lunatic Asylum* for Northumberland near Morpeth.
1859	*County of Sussex Asylum* in Haywards Heath, Sussex. This asylum served East Sussex following the Local Government Act of 1888.
1860	*The Stotfold Three Counties Asylum* later known as *Fairfield Hospital*, Bedfordshire. Replaced the former *Bedford Lunatic Asylum*.
1861	*Bristol City Asylum* replaced *St Peter's Hospital for Pauper Lunatics* in Bristol which had become unfit for purpose.
1862	*Cumberland and Westmorland Joint Lunatic Asylum* in Carlisle. Later known as *The Garlands Asylum*.
1863	*Broadmoor Criminal Lunatic Asylum* in Crowthorne, Berkshire. Later known as *Broadmoor Hospital*.
1863	*Second Dorset County Lunatic Asylum*. Later known as *Herrison Hospital*.
1865	*Burntwood Asylum* later to become *St Matthew's Hospital* near Lichfield was Staffordshire's second county asylum.

1867	*Surrey County Asylum* in Woking later known as *Brookwood Asylum* and *Brookwood Hospital*. This was the second county asylum for Surrey.
1869	*Leicester Borough Lunatic Asylum* at Humberstone, Leicestershire. This was a second county asylum for Leicestershire.
1869	*Newcastle upon Tyne Borough Lunatic Asylum* in Gosforth. Later known as *Newcastle upon Tyne City Lunatic Asylum*.
1870	*The Imbeciles Asylum*, Leavesden. This was one of the first institutions erected by the Metropolitan Asylums Board (1867) to administer care for some mental health disorders afflicting the sick poor in metropolitan London.
1870	*Ipswich Borough Mental Hospital* in Ipswich. Later known as *Ipswich Mental Hospital*.
1870	*Metropolitan Imbecile Asylum* at Caterham, Surrey. Later known as *Caterham Asylum.*
1870	*Moulsford Asylum in Moulsford* which is in the parish of Cholsey. This asylum was founded as a result of a union between Berkshire, Reading and Newbury for mental health purposes. The asylum was later known as *Fair Mile Hospital, Cholsey* and *Berkshire Mental Hospital*.
1871	*Cheshire County Asylum* also known as *Parkside Hospital* in Macclesfield was Cheshire's second asylum.
1871	*East Riding Lunatic Asylum* at Walkington, near Beverley. Later known as *Broadgate Hospital*.
1871	*Hereford Lunatic Asylum*. Later known as *The Hereford County and City Lunatic Asylum*. Provision for Herefordshire had from 1851 been at *The Joint Counties Lunatic Asylum* in Abergavenny. This was opened to serve the mid-Welsh counties of Monmouthshire, Brecknockshire and Radnorshire and had also included Herefordshire. The new asylum for Hereford was later known as *St Mary's Hospital.*
1872	*South Yorkshire Asylum*, Sheffield. Later known as *West Riding Asylum*, *Wadsley Mental Hospital* and *Middlewood Hospital*.
1873	*Whittingham Hospital*, Preston. This was Lancashire's fourth county asylum.
1873	*Royal Albert Asylum for Idiots and Imbeciles of the Seven Northern Counties* in Lancaster, Lancashire. It became known as *The Royal Albert Asylum for the Care, Education and*

	Training of Idiots, Imbeciles and Weak-Minded children and Young Persons of the Northern Counties in 1884.
1875	*Kent County Lunatic Asylum*, Chartham, Kent. Also known as *Chartham Asylum*. Later known as *Kent County Mental Hospital*, then *St Augustine's Hospital*. This was the second asylum for the county of Kent.
1876	*Northampton County Lunatic Asylum* for pauper patients in Upton, Northampton. It was also known as *Berrywood*, and later called *St Crispin Hospital*.
1877	*Banstead Asylum* in Banstead, Surrey. This was the third county asylum for Middlesex.
1878	*Darenth Asylum and Schools* in Dartford, Kent. Opened for 500 children with learning disabilities. Later known as *Darenth Industrial Training Colony*, then *Darenth Park Hospital*.
1879	*Portsmouth Lunatic Asylum* in Portsmouth.
1880	*Nottingham Borough Asylum* also known as *Mapperley Hospital*.
1882	*Birmingham Borough Asylum* in Rednal, Worcestershire. Also known as *Rubery Hill Hospital*.
1882	*Third Surrey County Pauper Lunatic Asylum* near Coulsdon. Also known as *Cane Hill*.
1883	*Hull Borough Asylum* in Hull, East Yorkshire
1885	*Gloucestershire County Asylum* later known as *Coney Hill Hospital*, Gloucester. This was the second county asylum for Gloucestershire.
1885	*Holloway Sanatorium*, Virginia Water, Surrey. An asylum for the care and treatment of the insane of the upper and middle classes.
1886	*Exeter City Lunatic Asylum*, officially opened as *The Exeter Asylum for the Insane*. Also known as the *Digby Hospital*, Exeter.
1888	*Derby Borough Lunatic Asylum* in Derby.
1888	*West Riding Asylum* in Ilkley. Later known as *Menston Mental Hospital*.
1891	*Plymouth Borough Asylum* in Ugborough, Ivybridge. Later known as *Blackadon Asylum*.
1892	*Tone Vale Hospital* near Taunton, Somerset was the second county asylum for Somerset. It was renamed *The Western Joint Asylum (Tone Vale)* in 1897.

1893	*Fifth London County Council Pauper Lunatic Asylum* in Woodford Bridge, Essex. Later known as *Claybury Asylum* and *Claybury Mental Hospital.*
1895	*Sunderland Borough Asylum* near Ryhope. Later known as *Cherry Knowle Asylum,* then *Cherry Knowle Hospital.*
1896	*Isle of Wight County Asylum.* The Isle of Wight became a separate county in 1890 and as a result needed its own asylum instead of sending patients to Hampshire which had been their previous practice. This asylum was later known as *Whitecroft Hospital.*
1897	*City of London Lunatic Asylum* near Dartford, Kent. Later known as *City of London Mental Hospital* and *Stone House Hospital.*
1897	*West Sussex County Asylum* at Graylingwell in Chichester. This asylum was built when the county of Sussex split into administrative areas following the Local Government Act of 1888. East and West Sussex became separate from each other as a result.
1898	*The Heath Asylum* in Bexley. Later known as *London County Asylum*, Bexley and *Bexley Asylum.*
1898	*Middlesbrough County Asylum* in Middlesbrough. Later known as *Middlesbrough Borough Asylum*, *Cleveland Asylum* and *Middlesbrough Mental Hospital.*
1899	*Cheddleton County Mental Asylum* later known as *St Edward's Hospital* near Leek. This was Staffordshire's third county asylum.
1899	*Hertfordshire County Asylum*, St Albans. Later known as *Hertfordshire County Mental Hospital*, then *Hill End Hospital.*
1899	*Sixth London County Asylum* in Epsom, Surrey. Also known as *The Manor Asylum*, *The Manor Certified Institution*, *Manor Mental Hospital.*

Chapter 5

Welsh Asylums in the
Nineteenth Century

In the late eighteenth century, Thomas Arnold (1742–1816) published his two volume *Observations on the Nature, Kinds, Causes and Prevention of Insanity*. Arnold qualified as a Doctor of Medicine at the University of Edinburgh in 1766, but spent the majority of his life in Leicester where he was the owner of one of the largest private madhouses in Britain. He was also physician of the new Leicester Lunatic Asylum. He stated that insanity, particularly of the melancholy kind, had previously been thought to be more prevalent in England than in any other country in Europe – although he did assert that there were instances of it in France. His work was both a mixture of national pride and anti-French prejudice as he attempted to prove that cases of insanity were more abundant in a country where 'the desire, and prospect, of acquiring riches, or the acquisition of them' made individuals more susceptible to insanity. He made a direct comparison between the state of lunacy in England and France and the conditions in both Scotland and Wales, which he described as 'neither opulent nor luxurious … but poorer and less cultivated areas.' He was of the firm opinion that as a result, insanity in these areas was very rare.

Perhaps Arnold's view was correct in some respects. Sir Andrew Halliday (1782–1839), who also qualified in medicine at the University of Edinburgh and became the Royal Physician to William IV and then to Queen Victoria, published *A General View of the present state of Lunatics and Lunatic Asylums in Great Britain and Ireland* following the *County Asylums Act* of 1828. He discovered that at this time there were only thirty-eight insane patients in institutional confinement in Wales, fourteen of whom were in Haverfordwest, Pembrokeshire. This was a very insignificant number and, on face value, appeared to confirm Arnold's opinion.

On closer examination, however, Halliday estimated the total number of insane and came to the conclusion that in the Principality of Wales in 1829, there were 153 lunatics and 763 idiots. He suspected that the actual numbers were likely to be in excess of this as many parishes had failed to complete a documentary return of their insane. He was convinced that very few of these individuals were in a proper place of refuge.

In 1829 the population of Wales was estimated at about 820,000. Judging from Halliday's figures, this suggested that one in every 800 people was suffering from a form of mental health disorder. Halliday was intrigued by this figure but determined that Wales, like Scotland, had a large proportion of its population living in agricultural districts. He concluded from this that 'hard labour and low diet may have an influence on offspring propagated by them increasing the numbers of idiotism.'

Regardless of the poor conditions and lack of provision for the mentally ill in Wales, there was only one county funded pauper asylum until 1844, despite the Acts of Parliament of 1808 requiring each county to build a place of refuge for their insane. In 1824 a small asylum opened in Haverfordwest. The asylum was housed in the former town gaol. In 1838 the Earl of Cawdor and other county magistrates visited the asylum and, appalled at what they found, requested the Home Office to carry out an inspection. This was done in November of the same year and the subsequent report declared that 'the asylum was unfit for purpose, and that the erection of another building more appropriate was imperatively called for.'

In 1843, the Lunacy Commissioners of England and Wales led by Lord Ashley again inspected the condition of Haverfordwest borough asylum and a report dated 8 September 1843 described the conditions in the asylum as 'much improved in both management and comfort … No person was under mechanical restraint, the patients were kindly treated but it was regrettable that no means of regular employment was provided.'

In an address to the House of Commons in 1844, Ashley made a point of singling out the asylum at Haverfordwest and, for dramatic effect to further his campaign for general improved asylum conditions in England and Wales, described the lunatic poor of Wales as 'too often treated as no man of feeling would treat his dog – they were kept in outhouses – chained – wallowing in filth and without firing for years [with no fire to provide warmth].' The acting magistracy of Pembrokeshire admitted that the existence of 'abuses and neglects' was undeniable and action to improve the system had been taken, however, they were concerned that their own Member of Parliament had not countered Ashley's allegations.

In the same address to the House of Commons, Ashley stated that following the Poor Law returns of 1843, it was revealed that there were 1,177 pauper lunatics in Wales. Of these, thirty-six were in English asylums, forty-two were in English licensed houses, ninety were in Union workhouses and a small number were in the lunatic asylum at Haverfordwest. The remainder were either kept at home, lodged with friends, or allowed to wander freely without supervision. Ashley further asserted that those who had been sent to English asylums were often done so when both their mental and physical condition had deteriorated to a very poor level. In order to illustrate this, he provided an example from an area of Brecon.

> *On 28 November 1843, Ann Abney was sent to the Hereford asylum from near Brecon. She died on 30 January 1844; she was in such a shocking state that the proprietor wished not to admit her. She had been kept chained in the crouching position, her knees were forced up to her chin, and she sat wholly upon her heels and hips, and considerable excoriation had taken place where her knees pressed against her stomach. She could not move about and was generally maniacal. When she died it required very considerable dissection to get her passed into her coffin.*

The Lunacy Commissioners recommended that a purpose built asylum to cater for the mentally ill of the southern counties of Wales should be erected, but no agreement to this proposal could be reached due to the likely extensive costs of such an enterprise.

During this period a privately licensed asylum opened at Vernon House, Briton Ferry, Neath in South Wales. Owned by Robert Valentine Leach, an advertisement announcing the establishment appeared in *The Welshman* newspaper on 17 November 1843. This asylum was primarily used by the county of Glamorgan. As a private asylum, however, the proprietor could charge what he wished and the Cardiff Union began to send their pauper insane to the County of Somerset Asylum at Wells in England, which was a considerably cheaper option. In 1857, there were 235 lunatics resident at Briton Ferry of whom twenty-four were private patients.

In North and Mid Wales, those requiring asylum admission were sent to their nearest English asylum, which was generally either the County Asylum of Cheshire at Chester, or the County Asylum of Gloucestershire at Gloucester. Some patients were also sent to smaller private 'madhouses' in Liverpool. This situation was far from ideal as many of the Welsh patients were unable to speak English and were, therefore, increasingly confused away from all that was familiar to them. Dr Samuel Hitch (1800–81), medical superintendent of Gloucester Lunatic Asylum wrote a letter to the editor of *The Times* about this matter and a copy of it also appeared in the *North Wales Chronicle* on 18 October 1842. His letter stated:

> *On being doomed to an imprisonment amongst strange people, and an association with his fellow men whom he is prohibited from holding communion with, nothing can exceed his misery; himself unable to communicate or to receive communications; harassed by events which he cannot make known, and appealed to by sounds which he cannot comprehend he becomes irritable and irritated ... This will probably be the only explanation that can ever be given how it passed into a proverb in English asylums that 'the Welshman is the most turbulent patient whenever he happens to become an inmate'.*

The first Welsh census that contained information about the language spoken by its inhabitants was in 1891. However, even at that stage, it was seen that ninety-three per cent of the population of Anglesey, Caernarfonshire and Merionethshire spoke Welsh with seventy per cent of the inhabitants having no English language. The further away people lived from the English border, the less likely they were to speak the language. Therefore, for the western counties of North Wales, the need for an asylum that provided care in an environment they understood was paramount.

In 1844 the five northern Welsh counties of Flintshire, Denbighshire, Merionethshire, Caernarfonshire and Anglesey came to an agreement to mutually fund an asylum at Denbigh in Denbighshire to cater for their mentally ill population. Montgomeryshire had also taken part in the early discussions but chose instead to continue to send its pauper lunatics to the English county of Shropshire for care. Anglesey and Caernarfonshire joined the venture late in the negotiations for the Denbigh asylum because they were using a facility called Haydock Lodge Asylum in Lancashire for their insane. Haydock Lodge was a private madhouse run by a former assistant Poor Law Commissioner called Charles Mott. Mott had engaged two Welsh-speaking nurses to work at the asylum for the benefit of the new patients expected from Wales. A description from its prospectus issued in 1845 describes it as follows:

> *The noble modern mansion stands within a spacious park, secluded from the public sight, and is connected with suitable attached and detached buildings, and large walled gardens, surrounded by about 370 acres of land, in a ring fence, affording facilities for recreation, healthful and interesting employment, superior to those attainable in any similar Asylum in England, – or indeed in Europe.*
>
> *The Establishment is conducted upon the system of non-restraint and kind moral-treatment so successfully employed by Dr. Conolly, and now followed at the Hanwell Middlesex County Asylum, forming a most gratifying contrast with the cruel and disgraceful treatment Pauper Lunatics were formerly subject to.*

In 1844 Dr Owen Owen Roberts, a medical practitioner from Bangor sent a patient, the Reverend Evan Richards, vicar of Llanwnda and Llanfaglen to Haydock Lodge because his family were concerned about his loss of mental power. As news began to emerge from other returning Welsh patients about neglect and cruelty occurring at the asylum, Roberts recommended to Reverend Richards' family that he should be removed. The medical condition of the vicar on his arrival home reached both the local and national press. On 20 June 1846 *The Caernarfon and Denbigh Herald* and *North and South Wales Independent* reported that:

> *Dr Roberts was shocked to find, upon a personal examination, the clearest proofs of shameful neglect and cruel treatment; that his body was covered with bruises, scars, and discolorations; that one of his toes was severely crushed; that one of his ears was as if it had been all but pulled off; and that his clothes were filthy and disgusting in the extreme.*

News of this case, and a petition by Dr Owen Owen Roberts, led to an enquiry by the Lunacy Commissioners, which resulted in Mott losing his position at Haydock Lodge. This situation heightened the fears of a similar situation occurring elsewhere for the insane of Caernarfon and Anglesey and as a result, both decided to join the Denbigh scheme.

The Reverend Richards clearly recovered from his experience because the 1851 census shows that he continued in his position as the vicar of Llanwnda and Llanfaglen parish where he was living with his wife Jane, a curate named Hugh Roberts, and three domestic servants. Without doubt, Richards was treated badly but the intervention of his doctor prevented others from Caernarfonshire being treated in the same way.

On 14 November 1848, the Clerk at the new asylum at Denbigh, John Robinson, wrote to the Board of Guardians at Bangor and Beaumaris Union to inform them that 'we are now in a position to receive as many patients as you may wish to send in.' The patients that were still being treated at Haydock Lodge could therefore be transferred immediately.

The asylum at Denbigh had cost the five northern counties over £23,000, but when constructed was able to accommodate about 200 people. As well as the patients previously treated at Haydock Lodge, many of its first patients were those already in the care of the asylums at Chester and Gloucester. The county approached Dr John Conolly, the resident physician at the Middlesex County Asylum at Hanwell, to

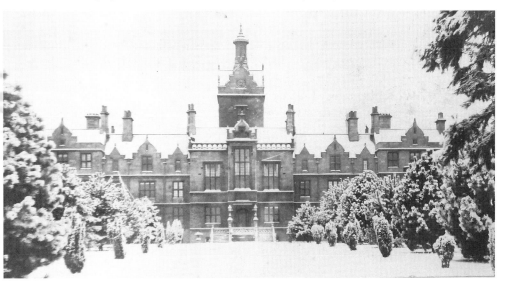

Denbigh Asylum, Wales. With permission from Denbighshire Archives.

recommend a suitable candidate as medical officer; George Turner Jones was appointed and sent to Gloucester Asylum for instruction. One of the main considerations of the committee responsible for the staffing at Denbigh was that the staff were Welsh speaking, which was considered highly important for the care of their patients. The asylum staff were recruited locally and therefore Welsh was their first language. As a result, despite being regulated under English law, the establishment became very much a Welsh institution. The asylum at Denbigh closed in 1995.

At a similar time (1851) The Joint Counties Lunatic Asylum in Abergavenny was opened to serve the mid Welsh counties of Monmouthshire, Herefordshire, Brecknockshire and Radnorshire. Prior to this date, patients from these four counties needing asylum care were occasionally sent to the small asylum at Whitchurch in Herefordshire, but, as in North Wales, were generally cared for within their community. The recommendations for the erection of a new asylum had been made at the Herefordshire Quarter Sessions in April 1846. The decision for a joint county enterprise was undertaken because no single county had more than fifty-five pauper lunatics requiring asylum care in the 1840s, and Breconshire and Radnorshire had considerably less than this number. In order to defray the expense of four separate buildings, one building serving all four counties was considered the best arrangement. During these sessions it was suggested that the counties of Carmarthenshire, Cardiganshire, Pembrokeshire and Glamorganshire adopt a similar practise and build a four counties asylum in Carmarthen as this was the centrical site.

The Joint Counties Lunatic Asylum in Abergavenny was initially designed to accommodate 250 patients but was later enlarged as the need for provision expanded. This asylum closed in 1996.

Following the recommendations of the Lunacy Commissioners and the encouragement of the Mid Wales Asylum Committee, in 1847, the counties of Cardiganshire, Carmarthenshire, Glamorgan and Pembrokeshire, agreed to build a four counties asylum. Glamorgan had deliberated over its decision to join the other counties as some felt it merited an asylum of its own. A site at Danycraig, Swansea in Glamorgan with accommodation for 350 patients was chosen because Glamorgan had the largest population and also good rail links thanks to the South Wales Railway. This asylum continued to be used until 1856 when the joint committee for the four counties was dissolved.

The Glamorgan County Lunatic Asylum at Angelton, Bridgend, opened in 1864 – it was managed by a committee of visitors appointed by the Quarter Sessions. Accommodation for 350 patients was initially provided, but soon proved inadequate.

Slater's Trade Directory of 1880 provides a description of the asylum at Angelton and allows us to see that it had:

> *A church which will accommodate about 250 patients; on the south side is the asylum farm; the dining hall adjoins the kitchen and is a lofty room about 80 feet long by 40 feet wide; the grounds cover about 14 acres of the estate, which consists in all of about 60 acres. It is calculated to accommodate over 600 patients, and is said to be the largest in South Wales. The river Ogmore runs through the grounds, which are beautifully laid out and planted, and its banks afford pleasant walks for the inmates.*

In 1887, a new building two miles away from Angelton was erected at Parc Gwyllt in Bridgend. The two establishments were connected to each other by telephone for ease of communication. *The Weekly Mail* published comments from the medical superintendent, Dr Henry Turnbull Pringle, in February 1887 in which he described his beliefs on the causes of insanity in the county. In many respects his views coincided with those of both Arnold and Halliday writing earlier the same century.

> *Compared with other counties in England and Wales, Glamorgan stands most favourably, there being only five other whose ratio of pauper lunatics to general population is slightly smaller. A considerable number of counties have to provide for a half more lunatics than Glamorganshire, and a few even double the number to the population. I believe this to be owing to its being an industrial county which offers great facilities to the more enterprising of the labourers from agricultural districts, who, attracted by high wages, make it their home and contract marriages, which, being mixed, tend to the production of a more healthy race than when, as in a stagnant agricultural district, there is a limited choice. This, at any rate, is the first effect, although eventually pursuits such as those of colliers and miners, tend to dwarf and deteriorate their descendants.*

A year after the new asylum in Glamorgan was built, a joint counties asylum was agreed for Carmarthenshire, Cardigan and Pembrokeshire at Carmarthen in south Wales. This asylum was opened in 1865 and had room for 212 patients. One of the first patients to be admitted, a man called Davies from Aberystwyth (described as a dangerous lunatic) succeeded in escaping from the asylum in the year that it opened but was re-apprehended the same day.

By January 1867 there were 174 lunatics resident in the Carmarthen Asylum and additional construction work for the benefit of the patients had been recommended. Again there was indecision and deliberations about funding and patient costs were increased from 12s to 14s a week which made them among the most expensive county-funded asylums in the country. Glamorgan however, was charging the same amount at the same time. It was thought that the running costs were greater because other asylums were more self-sufficient and could therefore charge less per patient. This amount was reduced in March 1869 to 11s 1d as the asylum was in a far better financial position. In the same year the northern counties asylum at Denbigh charged 8s 2d for pauper patients and 42s 6d for private patients and the mid-counties asylum at Abergavenny charged 9s for pauper patients.

Whilst funding in Carmarthen continued to be discussed, it was noted in 1869 that there remained within the three counties 420 lunatics in receipt of parish relief or lodged with their families. These individuals had not been sent to the asylum as for the main part, they were considered to be imbeciles and idiots who were harmless and in many cases were performing some useful activity within their communities. It was noted that asylum provision had never been intended for these people and that it was more beneficial for both them and the authorities to maintain their upkeep in their parishes. At this point the asylum had 232 patients, 114 men and 118 women and as such was operating above its intended capacity. It was clearly urgent that additional space be provided by a continuation of the building programme. The asylum was increased in size from 1869, and by 1876 was able to accommodate 390 patients divided into an allocated number for each individual county with 165 allocated to Carmarthenshire, 120 for Pembrokeshire and 105 for Cardigan.

The Royal Commission on the Ancient and Historical Monuments of Wales provides a detailed description of the site, which was closed in 2002.

This is a vast Italianate complex, generally three storey. The walls are of local stone with Bath stone dressings and have an inner brick skin. The roofs are generally hipped. It is set in extensive landscaped grounds. There is a grandiose central block including offices, the great dining hall and the original chapel. It is flanked by separate men's and women's ward ranges. These are broken by day room pavilions and infirmary blocks projecting into the segregated exercise yards or gardens. Great Italianate water towers with steep pyramid roofs rise over each wing. Behind the men's wards were workshops, the women being provided with a laundry. A remarkably forceful new chapel was built on the north side of the hospital in 1883-9. It was financed by the profits from private patients and patients provided the labour. A detached hospital for infectious diseases stands within the grounds to the west.

The following is a list of asylums built in Wales during the nineteenth century as a result of the 1808 County Asylums Act. These asylums were predominantly built for the pauper insane.

Year	Name and location of establishment
1847	*United Counties Lunatic Asylum* at Danycraig, Swansea in Glamorgan.
1848	*North Wales Counties Lunatic Asylum* in Denbigh, Denbighshire. Also known as *North Wales Counties Mental Hospital.*
1851	*Joint Counties Lunatic Asylum* in Abergavenny. Also known as *Monmouthshire Lunatic Asylum* and *Pen-y-Fal Hospital.*
1864	*Glamorgan County Lunatic Asylum* at Angelton, Bridgend.
1865	*The United Lunatic Asylum for Cardigan*, Carmarthen, Glamorgan and Pembroke in Job's Well, Carmarthen. Also known as *St David's.*
1887	*Parc Gwyllt Asylum* in Bridgend.

Chapter 6

Scottish Asylums in the Nineteenth Century

The Royal Hospital at Montrose was the first asylum for the insane to be established in Scotland and the first to be granted a Royal Charter. A Royal Charter was a formal document issued by the sovereign to establish significant organisations and institutions including hospitals, universities and professional bodies; the charter granted certain rights and powers. The asylum at Montrose was founded in 1781 by Mrs Susan Carnegie née Scott of Charleton near Montrose (1744–1821) and obtained its charter in 1810 as The Montrose Lunatic Asylum, Infirmary and Dispensary. There were another six chartered asylums in Scotland – the Royal Asylums of Aberdeen (opened in 1800); Dundee (1820); Edinburgh (1813); Glasgow (1814); James Murray's Royal Asylum in Perth (1827), and The Crichton Institution at Dumfries (1839).

These establishments were charitable foundations funded through philanthropic donations, public subscriptions and legacies. As such they were managed by private committees usually consisting of the 'trustees of dispositions in trust' or by local dignitaries and landed gentry, who had little or no medical input.

The original Aberdeen Lunatic Asylum was founded in 1800. It was financed through royalties from the eight-volume treatise on dance, *Sketches Relative to the History and Theory of Dancing,* written by the city's dancing master and musician, Francis Peacock (1723–1807). It opened in November 1800 at Clerkseat near Aberdeen, providing twelve cells for lunatics. In its first eighteen months, twenty-seven patients were admitted. By 1818 the asylum had sixty-three patients.

The Royal Edinburgh Asylum was established by Dr Andrew Duncan (1744–1828), Professor of the Theory of Medicine at the University of Edinburgh. Duncan was influenced in his desire to improve asylum conditions following the death of his friend, the Scottish poet Robert Fergusson (1750–74), who died in mysterious circumstances in the public bedlam, Darien House, in Edinburgh in 1774 after sustaining a head injury.

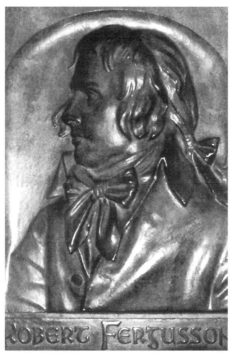

Memorial plaque to Robert Fergusson, St Giles Cathedral, Edinburgh. Photograph by Kathryn Burtinshaw, 2016.

Duncan had advocated that a properly designed, purpose built lunatic asylum should be established in Edinburgh as early as 1792 when he was President of the Royal College of Physicians in Edinburgh. Several difficulties were placed in Duncan's way – a Royal Charter was not granted until 1807, yet the asylum at Morningside did not open until 1813. The Royal Edinburgh Asylum was the only chartered asylum to receive any public funding – the asylum was awarded £2,000 from the sale of estates forfeited to the government of Great Britain following the crushing of Bonnie Prince Charlie's Jacobite rebellion of 1745 at the Battle of Culloden.

The original Glasgow Lunatic Asylum opened in 1814 in the Cowcaddens district of Glasgow but did not obtain its Royal Charter until 1824, when it became the Glasgow Royal Lunatic Asylum. Due to overcrowding it relocated to a much larger institution at Gartnavel in 1843. The new premises were designed to allow segregation by patients' gender and social class and were forward-thinking in their efforts to provide activities for their patients. In 1845 the asylum published *Gartnavel Minstrel* – the first publication written and edited by a hospital patient, J.R. Adam. It was dedicated to the Lord Provost of Glasgow and commended the work of Dr Hutcheson, medical superintendent of Gartnavel.

James Murray founded the Murray Royal Lunatic Asylum at Perth after inheriting a fortune in 1809 from his half-brother, a rich merchant in India, who drowned in a storm in a voyage home. James Murray left two-thirds of his estate for the purpose of establishing an asylum in his native Perth. Subsequently, the Murray Royal Hospital, designed by the architect William Burn (1789–1870), opened in 1827 with accommodation for eighty patients; it was a grand neo-classical building set in a pleasant open hillside site. The Perth Asylum was designed 'so that the meanest patient could be well fed and clothed, and those amongst the higher classes who could pay for it were lodged and cared for as they could be in a palace.' The aim was to provide a stable, homely and safe environment avoiding 'any gloomy appearance of confinement'. Although the asylum was established through funding from a legacy, it was maintained through public subscriptions donated by the generosity of the people of Perth.

The Dundee Lunatic Asylum was established as part of the Dundee Infirmary and was supported by voluntary contributions from 1810 onwards. The foundation stone was laid on 3 September 1812 and a parchment roll was buried with the foundation stone and inscribed:

To Restore the Use of Reason, to Alleviate Suffering and Lessen Peril where Reason cannot be Restored, the Dundee Lunatic Asylum was erected by Public Contribution.

The asylum was granted a Royal Charter in 1819 and formally opened in 1820 in Albert Street, Dundee.

The Crichton Royal Hospital was the last and the grandest of

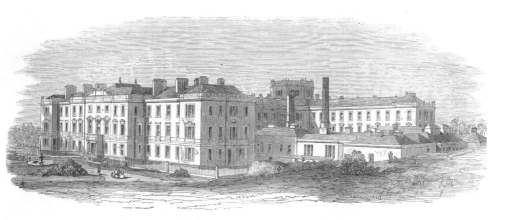

Crichton Royal Institute, Dumfries. Illustrated London News, 1872.

Scotland's royal asylums. It was founded in 1838 through the benevolence of Elizabeth Crichton née Grierson, of Friar's Carse (1779–1862) and other trustees, funded by a legacy of her late husband Dr James Crichton (1765–1823), erstwhile physician to the Governor General of India who had made a fortune in the service of the East India Company as a trader in China and India. Elizabeth Crichton had heard about Dr W.A.F. Browne's work at Montrose and his publication of *What asylums were, are and ought to be* and held him in great esteem and 'high reputation'. She endowed around £100,000 for the building of an asylum in Dumfries for 120 patients. It was a luxurious private establishment designed for the upper classes and opened on 5 June 1839. It had its own theatre, natural history museum, billiard room and an extensive library for the recreation and amusement of its residents. By more than doubling his salary at the Montrose Asylum, Elizabeth Crichton persuaded W.A.F. Browne to be the first medical superintendent of this new, first-rate, prestigious asylum. There, Browne could develop and advance his ideas of occupational and art therapy – a post he readily accepted.

At this time there was only one charitable public asylum for paupers in Scotland, at Elgin in Morayshire. The Elgin Pauper Asylum opened in 1835, with the land being donated by St Giles' Church and its annual funding coming from public contributions and rates. The asylum was also known as Bilbohall Hospital and was founded by the managers of Dr Gray's Hospital in the town. Not only was it the earliest asylum built specifically for paupers in Scotland, it was also the only one established before the 1857 *Lunacy (Scotland) Act*.

The chartered asylums were all situated in cities or populous towns and there was a clear lack of provision for the mentally unwell in the remote areas of the Highlands and Islands of Scotland. The chartered asylums did admit a limited number of pauper lunatics, charging the patient's parish of origin maintenance fees of between £21 and £28 a year to cover the costs of food, clothing, bedding, fuel, lighting, and the attendants' and servants' salaries and wages. However, for economic reasons, the parishes often sought cheaper accommodation for their insane parishioners in lunatic wards attached to hospitals, or in licensed madhouses, where the standard of treatment was uncertain.

These licensed madhouses were greatly overcrowded, unhygienic, and did nothing to promote recovery. In the mid-nineteenth century their proprietors received £20 to £22 per annum for accepting pauper lunatics. Many sought to accommodate as many lunatics as possible at the lowest possible expenditure aiming for large profits. These houses were scantily furnished; the cooking, sanitary and washing facilities were poor; there was a lack of heating and ventilation; clothing and bedding provision was minimal; there was little if any opportunity for exercise or even 'airing' of inmates; and, no arrangements were made for the proper treatment of those suffering from sickness or disability. These institutions literally stank, and were harbours of infectious disease. Instrumental methods of restraint with manacles, leg-locks, straps and straight-jackets were widely used both to prevent escape, and to avoid lunatics attacking attendants or other patients. These methods were often resorted to because of an inadequate number of attendants. There are reports of manacles being used to fasten the arms behind the back, and also to rings fixed in the walls. Mortality rates in the licensed madhouses were high, particularly in winter when exposure to the cold was an additional problem. Profit was prioritised over the welfare and benefit of the patients.

It was clear that patients placed in the Royal or chartered asylums achieved a far more favourable outcome than patients placed within licensed madhouses. Subsequently Thomas Hamilton (1780–1858), as Lord Binning of Tyninghame, Member of Parliament, proposed a 'Scotch Lunatic Asylum Bill' before Parliament in 1818 to erect a new system of four district lunatic asylums throughout Scotland for pauper lunatics, each with their own district commissioners based on the model of the English 1808 *County Asylums Act*. The proposed revenue for the scheme was to come from rates – this was unpopular with the heritors (land owners) who paid rates and unfortunately this Bill was opposed.

The asylums soon filled beyond capacity and extra accommodation was required. At Edinburgh a new building, West House, was built in 1837 alongside the existing asylum at Morningside. It became the main Royal Edinburgh Asylum, and the original building, renamed East House, was subsequently used exclusively for private patients. At Montrose, with the number of patients exceeding 200, a much larger replacement asylum was built at Sunnyside between 1855 and 1858 and the former buildings were sold to the army. By the end of 1860 there were 373 patients in residence there.

Asylum buildings were designed to segregate males from females; those at the 'lower ranks' of society from the 'higher ranks'; and, in each division by mental state ('ordinary', 'frantic', 'convalescent' and 'incurable').

In 1857 there were 2,172 patients in the seven chartered asylums and the pauper asylum at Elgin. There were 5,240 lunatics elsewhere in Scotland, mostly in unlicensed private houses. There is no doubt that reform was overdue. Dorothea Dix's visit to Scotland in 1855 (see Chapter 3) was very influential in the Scottish reforms and she certainly had the celebrity support of Lord Shaftesbury, the Duke of Argyll and Sir George Grey, the Home Secretary. The 1857 *Lunacy (Scotland) Act* divided Scotland into administrative Lunacy Districts each with a district board required 'to provide for the building of District Asylums for the reception of pauper lunatics and to ensure the proper care and treatment of lunatics generally, whether placed in asylums, or left in private houses under the care of relatives or strangers'. Whereas the chartered asylums had catered principally for private patients and accommodated a few paupers, the new District Asylums were specifically intended to cater for paupers or those belonging to the low-income labouring classes who were not strictly paupers. By 1859 Scotland had been divided into twenty-one Lunacy Districts. The Act made no provision for mental disability in the form of 'idiots' or 'imbeciles' (see Chapter 13).

The most important administrative outcome of the 1857 Act was the creation of a General Board of Commissioners in Lunacy. This General

Board succeeded in asylum development and the establishment of some form of public institution for the care of the mentally ill in most parts of Scotland. Nineteen District Asylums and two Parochial Asylums were established, mainly in areas where there was a lack of provision for pauper lunatics (see table below). Private patients would continue to be accommodated in the chartered asylums. The District Boards were also responsible for the construction and management of the new asylums. They had to identify suitable sites, engage architects (often after a competition), provide costings, obtain approval from the General Board, and then manage the building process. Once the asylum opened, the District Board was responsible for its day-to-day running, including the engagement and management of staff. District Boards were required to provide annual reports and accounts to the General Board.

Year	Name and location of establishment
1863	*Argyll & Bute District Asylum*, Lochgilphead, Argyllshire
1864	*Northern Counties District Asylum*, Craig Dunain, Inverness
1864	*Perth District Asylum*, Murthly, Perthshire
1865	*Banff District Asylum*, Banff, Banffshire
1866	*Ayrshire District Asylum*, Glengall, Ayrshire
1866	*Haddington District Asylum*, Haddington, East Lothian
1866	*Stirling District Asylum*, Larbert, Stirlingshire
1866	*Fife & Kinross District Asylum*, Stratheden, near Cupar, Fife
1869	*Roxburgh, Berwick & Selkirk District Asylum*, Melrose, Roxburghshire
1872	*Bothwell District Asylum*, Kirklands, Bothwell, Lanarkshire
1874	*Midlothian & Peebles District Asylum*, Rosslyn, Midlothian
1875	*Barony Parochial Asylum*, Woodilee, Lenzie, Dunbartonshire
1876	*Paisley & Johnston District Asylum*, Riccartsbar, Paisley, Renfrewshire
1876	*Greenock Poorhouse and Parochial Asylum*, Greenock, Renfrewshire
1877	*Dundee District Asylum, Liff, Dundee*, City of Dundee
1889	*City of Glasgow District Asylum for Pauper Lunatics*, Gartloch
1890	*Govan District Asylum*, Hawkhead, Govan, Renfrewshire
1895	*Lanark District Asylum*, Hartwood, Shotts, Lanarkshire

1898	*Edinburgh District Asylum*, Bangour, Uphall, West Lothian
1899	*Aberdeen District Asylum*, Kingseat, Aberdeen, City of Aberdeen
1909	*Renfrew District Asylum*, Dykebar, Paisley, Renfrewshire

Pauper Lunatic Asylums established in Scotland 1857–1909.

The asylum population increased throughout the nineteenth century. The later asylums were much larger than the earlier ones in order to accommodate greater numbers of patients. In the last quarter of the century many of the existing asylums were enlarged by the addition of new wings, recreation halls, outbuildings, hospital blocks, and sometimes churches or farm buildings. Kitchens and laundries were also expanded and improvements were made to inadequate water supplies, drainage and sanitary arrangements.

The case of the water supply for the Roxburgh District Asylum exemplifies the difficulties that Boards could have in getting local landowners to agree access to land and water sources. There was a prolonged drought in the south of Scotland in the summer of 1893. The Annual Report of 1894 stated that the water supply to the asylum:

> *... from all sources, good or bad, was quite insufficient. It was found necessary to discontinue the bathing of the patients to cease cleansing the floors, to restrict washing of clothes, to cut off the water in the lavatories during the greater part of the day, and to shut up many of the WCs; while, as regards risks from fire, the institution was reduced to a practically defenceless position.*

It took an Act of Parliament to enforce the compulsory purchase of twenty-seven acres of wasteland from the 6th Duke of Buccleuch to obtain sufficient water sources for the Roxburgh District Asylum. After years of fruitless negotiation, the *Roxburgh, Berwick, and Selkirk District Board of Lunacy (Water Supply) Act* of 1896 resolved the situation and in the 1898 Annual Report the asylum was 'now in possession of a supply of excellent water sufficient for its present requirements.'

Almost universally, the District Asylums in Scotland adopted Browne's moral approach to mental illness – through kindness, discipline, routines and the prescription of work. Browne firmly believed that cures

95

could be achieved through hard labour and keeping the mentally ill occupied in assisting with jobs within the asylum, or by working the land around the asylum. Therapeutic occupation through employment was seen as beneficial in two ways – it would prepare patients for their reintegration into society, and it could shorten their stay in the asylum by bringing forward their feelings of self-worth. A typical annual report by the medical superintendent of Roxburgh District Asylum in 1888 reported:

> *Much attention continues to be paid to the useful and healthy employment of the patients. For the men there is an unfailing supply of active and wholesome work in the cultivation of the gardens and improvements in the grounds. Others of the men are employed in the workshops as shoemakers, tailors, blacksmiths, joiners, masons, upholsterers &c. For the women employment has been found in the laundry, sewing-room, kitchen, and the wards.*

The Scottish asylums were quick to develop a system of 'boarding-out' by transferring harmless and incurable patients with a stable medical condition back into the community. This process was outlined by Dr John Carlyle Johnstone in 1887 as 'inoffensive unrecovered cases as no longer require asylum treatment [were removed] into private dwellings within the community either to family members or to strangers.' By doing so, this freed up space in overcrowded asylums – and was, in reality, an innovative nineteenth century method to address 'bed-blocking', which was a serious problem in the English asylums of the day. Boarding-out colonies developed throughout Scotland – the most well-known being that in the village of Kennoway in Fife where patients from Edinburgh were boarded out. Other colonies were established at Balfron in Stirlingshire, Aberfoyle in Perthshire, Loanhead in Midlothian, and on the Isle of Arran.

A leading article in the *British Medical Journal* in 1892 suggested that two distinct types of institutions were required – care homes for the chronic incurable cases and hospitals for the acutely mentally ill. At the end of the nineteenth century, detached hospital blocks were built at a number of Scottish asylums. They had a higher staffing level and were designed to cater for new admissions and patients with acute illnesses. Nevertheless, at the end of the nineteenth century the demand for places in the asylums had continued to increase and as a result asylums were stretched beyond capacity and remained overcrowded.

Chapter 7

Irish Asylums in the Nineteenth Century

PRIVATE ASYLUMS AND MADHOUSES

In 1805 when there were forty-five private madhouses in England there was only one in Ireland – the 'Cittadella' at Blackrock near Cork, established in 1799 by Dr William Saunders Hallaran, which catered predominantly for upper class patients. Hallaran was an established alienist, and was concurrently the visiting physician to the public lunatic asylum at Cork.

The Religious Society of Friends (the Quakers) established a private 'Retreat for Persons Afflicted with Disorders of the Mind in Ireland', which opened as The Bloomfield Retreat in Donnybrook Road in Dublin in 1812, capable of accommodating thirty patients. Bloomfield's philosophy was based on the ethos of moral treatment promoted by the Tuke family at The York Retreat in England (see Chapter 2). Bloomfield opened its doors to non-Quakers in 1821.

Another private asylum was opened at Farnham House, Finglas, County Dublin in 1814 but solely for the treatment of the upper and middle classes. It was established by Dr James Duncan, who had graduated from the Royal College of Surgeons of Edinburgh in 1805. His two sons, James Foulis Duncan (1812–95) and Nugent Booker Duncan (1813–84), both graduated in Medicine. Nugent assisted his father at Farnham. James graduated as Doctor of Medicine from the University of Dublin in 1847 and was consulting physician to the Adelaide Hospital in Dublin, and at one time President of the Royal College of Physicians. He resigned this post on his father's death in 1868 to succeed as proprietor and superintendent of Farnham. John Foulis Duncan became president of the Medico-Psychological Association in 1875.

As outlined in Chapter 2, the writer Jonathan Swift, author of *Gulliver's*

Travels, provided a legacy for the foundation of St Patrick's Hospital in Dublin, which opened in 1757 catering primarily for private patients in the early part of the century, as did the lunatic asylum at Cork. The number of private asylums in Ireland slowly increased in the first half of the nineteenth century. By 1844 there were fourteen registered private asylums in Ireland – seven of them in the Dublin area. However, with changes in legislation and the establishment of state funded asylums, the number of private asylums remained fairly low with only twenty registered in 1893.

PUBLIC ASYLUMS

By 1808 the Dublin house of industry provided for seventy-six 'maniacs requiring confinement and coercion'. In Clonmel there were thirty-six cells for lunatics in 1811, but many inmates 'lay naked in a yard on bundles of straw and those in the vicinity could hear their bellowing and hideous noise.' In reality, because there was no provision for the payment for transport to one of the lunatic wards in a house of industry, most lunatics in rural Ireland were committed to a local gaol. Those who were admitted to houses of industry were often required to make a lengthy and dreadful journey over the rough roads of the time. It was customary to tie them by the wrists to a cart and make them walk behind it to the workhouse. The situation began to improve following the 1817 Select Committee Enquiry discussed in Chapter 3.

At the start of the nineteenth century there was only public provision for 250 insane people in Ireland – ninety in Cork Lunatic Asylum (established 1789), 118 in the Dublin house of industry and the remainder in the Waterford and Limerick houses of industry. In addition, there were hundreds of insane people in gaols or bridewells. Most lunatics and idiots were 'at large' wandering the streets and the countryside, or confined in peasant cabins or outhouses. Several were vagrants or beggars and lived on the charity of others, pleading for food and shelter. Some were put on public display by their families outside churches and at fairs with the hope of provoking sympathy and receiving alms. Village idiots were the subject of public sport, being mocked by children and adults alike whereas maniacal 'furious' lunatics could be a genuine threat to a neighbourhood.

Richmond Asylum (later re-named St Brendan's Hospital) at Grangegorman, Dublin was opened in 1815 as the first national facility to receive and care for lunatics from all parts of Ireland and as such was the oldest public hospital in Ireland that catered for mental health disorders.

The governors of the Dublin house of industry together with the physician Dr Alexander Jackson (1767–1848), appointed there in 1795, obtained a government grant to establish a dedicated, purpose-built asylum adjacent to the workhouse. Richmond was named after the current Lord Lieutenant, Charles Lennox, 4th Duke of Richmond (1764–1819), and was initially built to accommodate 218 curable patients (including forty-two private patients), but on opening, it immediately received 170 lunatics directly from the house of industry in Dublin. Although there was a lay manager, Jackson became the asylum's first medical officer and, having previously taken a tour of English asylums, he advocated moral treatment rather than 'all the apparatus of chains, darkness and anodynes'. The establishment was intended for curable patients only – with incurable patients being looked after in a house of industry. Those seeking admission to the asylum had to be screened in the house of industry in order to place them in the appropriate institution. Asylum admission required a certificate of insanity signed either by a medical practitioner, a clergyman or a magistrate. Richmond Asylum soon filled well beyond capacity. This made it clear that far greater provision for lunatics in Ireland was necessary.

By 1817 St Patrick's Hospital, Dublin (Swift's Hospital), had fifty-three fee-paying 'boarders' (private patients) and ninety-six resident paupers paid for by voluntary donations and parliamentary grants. The fees charged to boarders varied from 30 to 100 guineas a year – those paying the maximum fee were allocated two rooms and a servant for their exclusive use.

The Irish government was quick to recognise that the provision of a network of public asylums for and across the whole country was essential, and did so as early as 1817 – it was not until 1845 before a similar requirement was acknowledged in England. Robert Peel (1788–1850), as Chief Secretary of Ireland 1812–1817, and the leading Irish Whig Sir John Newport (1756–1843) with support from Thomas Spring Rice, were instrumental in pursuing the legislative process leading to the 1817 *Asylums for Lunatic Poor (Ireland) Act* and the 1821 *Lunatic Asylums (Ireland) Act.* The Irish administration, essentially acting as the English government in Ireland, was empowered to impose the establishment of lunatic asylums countrywide from 1817. It was authorised to divide the country into suitable districts, to set the amount of each county's contribution to the asylum, to nominate the governors and establish a Board of Control to oversee the asylum system.

By 1830, however, only four new district asylums had been completed in Ireland: Armagh, Limerick, Derry, and Belfast (see table below). After 1830, Richmond Asylum was incorporated into the district asylum system by way of *The Richmond Lunatic Asylum Act* of 1830. A new district asylum was opened at Carlow in May 1832 to serve the counties of Carlow, Kildare, Wexford and Kilkenny. The Maryborough Asylum was opened in1833 to serve King's County (now County Offaly) and Queen's County (now County Laois), County Westmeath and County Longford. It later became Portlaoise Asylum.

Connaught District Lunatic Asylum, at Ballinasloe, County Galway was opened in 1833, initially for 150 curable patients serving counties Galway, Roscommon, Mayo, Sligo and Lethin – the province of Connaught – which had a population of 1,340,000 at that time. Asylums at Clonmel (1835) and Waterford (1835) opened shortly thereafter. When these asylums started taking patients, their Boards of Governors believed that they were moving forward with modern, progressive institutions for the treatment and recovery of curable lunatics. However, the asylums soon filled up with disruptive incurable lunatics and congenital idiots who were transferred from infirmaries, houses of industry and gaols. For example, the Minutes of the Board of Guardians of Connaught District Asylum of 7 May 1835 lamented that the asylum, built to accommodate 150 curable patients, was almost full within two years of opening. Of the146 patients in the asylum at that date:

> *eighty-six have been admitted from the several gaols of the Province who with a few exceptions have been Incurable, Epileptic or Idiotic and are therefore likely to remain in the asylum during life.*

The district asylums exceeded capacity soon after opening and by 1837 there were over 1,600 lunatics in these grossly overcrowded district institutions with over a further 1,500 people with mental health problems detained in gaols, houses of industry, or private asylums. One of the difficulties was that the Inspector General of Prisons for Ireland, Major Benjamin Blake Woodward (1769–1841), a qualified lawyer and the former Member of the Irish Parliament for Midleton in County Cork, was also Inspector of Asylums and pursued his own agenda. Woodward perceived asylums as a natural dumping ground for lunatics to aid the smooth running of his gaols where insane inmates could be disruptive.

He argued that legally, asylums had an obligation to accept patients from gaols by citing that 'the Commissioners of any lunatic asylum are empowered to receive of Idiots and Epileptics &c. a number not exceeding half of their establishment.'

Rules set out by the Privy Council of Ireland in 1843 stipulated that every asylum in Ireland had to provide both a Roman Catholic and a Presbyterian chaplain – neither of whom were required to live in the asylum. The asylums had to provide a chapel for a religious service every Sunday and on Good Friday and Christmas Day. A residence for the chaplains could be provided in the asylum grounds but this was not a legal requirement. Religious instruction was seen as part of moral therapy, although patients suffering from 'religious excitement' were only allowed to attend the services with special permission from the medical superintendent.

By 1845 there were only ten district asylums in existence scattered throughout Ireland providing just 1,300 places for lunatics. Other lunatics were looked after in a number of miserable and inadequate private asylums. At this time there were fourteen private licenced asylums in Ireland, seven of which were in Dublin including Farnham House at Finglas, three miles from Dublin Castle (see above).

The establishment of an Inspectorate of Lunacy in Ireland within the Chief Secretary's Office in 1846, dealing exclusively with lunatics, led to a review of the standards of care, the establishment of more asylums, and an increase in rates to pay for them. The first Inspector-General of Lunacy was Dr Francis White (1787–1859), medical superintendent of Richmond Asylum, appointed to the post on 1 January 1846. Sir John Nugent (1806–99), a medical graduate of Trinity College Dublin, joined him the following year. Together they held the responsibility for inspecting and reporting on all aspects of asylums and other institutions caring for the insane throughout Ireland. They generated a dominant influence on the evolution of the asylum system in Ireland. The management of asylums subsequently passed from lay supervisors to members of the medical profession. Like their contemporary English and Scottish colleagues, White and Nugent encouraged the development of moral values, emphasising kindness and comfort as the most effective therapy for the mentally ill. They secured the appointment of chaplains in district asylums. By the 1860s all of the district asylums had medically trained resident managers, known as medical superintendents, who could be either a physician or a surgeon. An independent doctor, known as a visiting physician or surgeon, usually a man of standing in his profession and of a different discipline to the medical superintendent, would advise on medical matters.

The Great Famine of 1845–52 caused by failure of the potato crop led to mass starvation and disease. During that time the population of Ireland fell by more than twenty per cent. Approximately one million people died and another million emigrated. The houses of industry filled up and the rate of insanity increased.

Between 1845 and 1853 the public asylums at Belfast, Carlow, Clonmel, Derry, Limerick, Maryborough, Richmond and Waterford were all extended, increasing the capacity for the number of patients. In 1851 there were 3,234 individuals resident in asylums. New asylums were opened at Mullingar; County Westmeath (1855); Cork and also at Killarney; Sligo; Omagh; and Kilkenny (see Table below). The new asylum at Cork, which opened in 1852 to replace the existing asylum attached to the house of industry, was called Eglinton Asylum, named after Archibald Montgomie (1812–61), 13th Earl of Eglinton, the then Lord Lieutenant of Ireland.

Before 1850, when the Central Criminal Lunatic Asylum was opened at Dundrum near Dublin, there was no special facility for criminal lunatics in Ireland. As in England and Wales at this time, insane individuals deemed to be criminals were held with other mentally ill patients in county asylums or in gaols.

The Omagh District Lunatic Asylum, opened in 1851, was initially built to accommodate 300 patients from the counties of Tyrone and Fermanagh. Its first resident physician was Dr Francis John West (d. 1880).

The Kilkenny Asylum, opened in 1852, was built to accommodate 150 patients from the city and county of Kilkenny. These patients had previously been in the catchment area of Carlow District Lunatic Asylum. By 1870 the asylum had 226 residents, rising to 243 in 1880, 320 in 1890 and 441 in 1900.

A further series of new district asylums was opened in the 1860s; they were typically large three-storey buildings situated on the outskirts of larger towns with land attached. The land was cultivated and farmed by the inmates, providing food for the institution. After 1866, Ballinasloe Asylum catered only for the counties of Galway and Roscommon. The new asylums were Castlebar; Letterkenny; Ennis; Enniscorthy; Downpatrick; and Monaghan (see Table below). Apart from Antrim

Asylum, which opened in 1899, no further asylums were built in the nineteenth century. In 1851 there were 3,234 individuals in Irish asylums. This number rose to 11,265 at the time of the 1891 census. By 1901 there were almost 17,000 inmates in twenty-two Irish asylums.

Throughout the last quarter of the nineteenth century there was concern that the incidence of mental illness in Ireland was increasing at a disproportionate rate compared to the rest of the United Kingdom. In 1884 it was reported that there were proportionally twice as many lunatics *per capita* in Ireland compared to England. Irish asylum doctors put this down to an accumulation of chronic cases in asylums. Other factors given in explanation were the high levels of emigration, poverty, intermarriage, and economic and political stress. Alcohol consumption was also deemed an 'exciting' cause of lunacy, with alcohol readily available due to the illicit distillation of *poitín*. Dietary changes were also blamed with a shift from porridge and potatoes to bread and tea. Strong, long-brewed tea was thought to be particularly 'exciting'.

Irish society appeared to accept state institutions providing social or medical care by means of workhouses and asylums. To the family, friends and neighbours of those committed, admission to an asylum removed their burden of care and any threat of violence, and presented the patient with a hope of cure. The asylum offered a place of safety, and a more comfortable environment than the workhouse or, in many cases, the home.

Throughout the nineteenth century the number of asylums continually grew and the existing asylums expanded. Whereas the populations of inmates in workhouses and prisons decreased, asylum populations perpetually increased. By 1901 there were almost 17,000 inmates in asylums originally planned for less than 5,000.

Year	Name and location of establishment
1815	*Richmond Asylum* (*St Brendan's*), Grangegorman, Dublin.
1825	*Armagh District Lunatic Asylum* (*St Luke's*), County Armagh (to accommodate 160 patients from Counties Tyrone, Donegal, Monaghan and Armagh).
1827	*Limerick Asylum*, County Limerick (to accommodate 150 patients from Counties Limerick, Clare and Kerry).
1829	*Derry District Asylum*, Londonderry, County Londonderry (to

	accommodate 120 patients from Counties Londonderry, Donegal and Tyrone).
1829	*Belfast District Lunatic Asylum*, Belfast (to accommodate 104 patients from Counties Antrim and Down).
1832	*Carlow Lunatic Asylum* (St Dympna's), Carlow, County Carlow (originally serving 100 patients from Counties Carlow, Kildare, Wexford and Kilkenny).
1833	*Maryborough District Lunatic Asylum*, Maryborough, County Laois (serving 170 patients from King's County and Queen's County, County Westmeath and County Longford).
1833	*Connaught District Asylum*, Ballinasloe, County Galway (serving 150 patients from Counties Galway, Roscommon, Mayo and Sligo [the province of Connaught]).
1835	*Clonmel District Asylum*, County Tipperary (60 beds).
1835	*Waterford District Asylum (St Otteran's)*, Waterford, County Waterford (100 beds).
1851	*Omagh District Asylum*, County Tyrone (to accommodate 300 patients from Counties Tyrone and Fermanagh).
1852	*Cork Asylum*, County Cork (replacing the original private Eglinton Asylum, to accommodate 500 patients).
1852	*Killarney District Asylum* (St Finan's), County Kerry (220 beds).
1852	*Kilkenny*, County Kilkenny (to accommodate 152 patients from the City and County of Kilkenny who has previously been housed in *Carlow Asylum*).
1855	*Mullingar*, County Westmeath (563 beds).
1855	*Sligo Lunatic Asylum* (St Columba's), County Sligo (470 beds).
1866	*Castlebar District Lunatic Asylum* (St Mary's), County Mayo (260 beds).
1866	*Letterkenny Asylum* (St Conal's), County Donegal (300 beds).
1868	*Ennis Lunatic Asylum* (Our Lady's Hospital), County Clare (260 beds).
1868	*Enniscorthy Asylum*, County Wexford (patients were previously admitted to *Carlow Asylum*) (330 beds).
1869	*Downpatrick Asylum* (Downshire), County Down (300 beds).
1869	*Monaghan District Lunatic Asylum*, Monaghan, County Monaghan (250 beds).
1899	*Antrim Asylum* (Holywell), Antrim, County Antrim (400 beds).

Table of District Lunatic Asylums in Ireland

Chapter 8

The Channel Islands

The Channel Islands comprise a separate group of islands not incorporated as part of the United Kingdom, though enjoying the protection of the Crown. They are divided into two British Crown Dependencies, the Bailiwicks of Guernsey and Jersey. The former also includes the islands of Alderney, Sark and Herm. The Channel Islands were historically owned by the Duchy of Normandy, and passed to the English Crown when William the Conqueror became King of England in 1066. Many members of the population continue to speak French as their first language.

Laws passed by the States are given Royal Sanction by the Queen in Council. Crown interests are represented by Lieutenant Governors. As a result of this, Jersey and Guernsey had different lunacy laws from other countries within the United Kingdom in the nineteenth century.

Before official provision for the insane on the islands, many individuals with mental health problems were cared for within their family home. Those considered to be dangerous or too difficult to manage within a home environment, were locked in outhouses or other buildings to prevent them wandering unsupervised on the islands and were often poorly treated by their families. In many cases local communities were aware of these individuals but turned 'a blind eye' to this form of treatment, accepting it as satisfactory. However, once the British Government in Westminster learned about the actual circumstances of this provision, pressure was brought to bear on the respective islands to provide appropriate asylum care for their insane.

Jersey

As in Scotland and Wales, cost was an important consideration and acted as a deterrent from action being taken to provide a publically funded asylum. In Jersey, following an investigation into a case of pronounced neglect on an insane woman discovered by a visiting English cattle dealer in 1846 and highlighted to British authorities, it was estimated that the number of insane people on the island did not amount to more than fifty. Given this low number, the expense of constructing a purpose built asylum was not considered necessary.

Lunatics who had no one willing or able to care for them on the island of Jersey were sent to the General Hospital at St Helier because there was nowhere else for them to go. The hospital became a multi-functional establishment for the care of the sick, the reception of the poor and the incarceration of the insane. In 1847 the hospital housed thirty-eight lunatics and idiots. By 1852 this number had increased to forty-six, of whom fourteen were considered dangerous. The hospital committee requested the power to send lunatics who were dangerous to asylums in France or England in an attempt that this appropriate provision may facilitate their cure. The matter was referred to the Home Office who would not allow any British subject to be confined in a lunatic asylum beyond British control. It was decided that those affected by mental derangement should not be sent to France despite the benefits this would provide to French speaking Jersey patients.

By 1861 there was a private asylum on the island called 'The Bagatelle Retreat' run by Isaac Pothecary. Pothecary had a scandalous reputation, having previously run an asylum called Grove Place in Hampshire, England with a partner, Dr William Symes. On 8 April 1854 *The Hampshire Telegraph and Sussex Chronicle* published a letter from the Secretary of the Lunacy Commissioners, which contained details of the lack of suitability of Grove Place and its owners as a place of care for the insane. The letter stated:

The Commissioners and Visitors have repeatedly noticed a want of warmth, a want of cleanliness, of clothing and bedding, a want of tables, seats, and other furniture, and an insufficient provision for the sick and infirm patients, also the bad state of the crib rooms, and generally that part of the premises occupied by the paupers. It will be observed also that the numbers allowed by the licence have repeatedly been exceeded, that the bath has been used as a punishment and not as a remedy for disease, and that the patients have repeatedly complained, and apparently with reason, of having been ill-treated by the attendants and others, and that the supervision of the Proprietors of the asylum has been (as indeed it must necessarily have been in order to allow of the existence of such numerous defects) extremely superficial, and that the want of substantial kindness and liberality towards their patients has been such as to prove their unfitness to have lunatic patients entrusted to their care.

Having been repeatedly criticised by the Lunacy Commissioners, in 1854 after six years at Grove Place, Pothecary and Symes dissolved their partnership and the asylum closed when the commissioners refused to renew their licence. By 1855 Pothecary was declared bankrupt and Symes had died, having been certified a lunatic himself. Pothecary moved to Jersey the same year, attempting to take with him the contents of Grove Place, which were due to be auctioned to pay his debts. The goods were recovered from the ship *Oracle* before it sailed from Southampton to Jersey.

However, as the Channel Islands did not fall under the same lunacy regulations as the rest of the United Kingdom, Pothecary was able to set up a private asylum in St Saviour. *The Hampshire Advertiser & Salisbury Guardian* briefly reported on 23 April 1859 that Pothecary had purchased 'Bagatelle' which he intended to convert into an asylum. The 1861 census reveals that there were twenty boarders resident in the establishment, several of whom were described as 'gentlewomen'. Two of the boarders, Mary Ann and Charlotte Blandford who were middle-aged spinsters, were recorded on the 1851 census living with Pothecary – at that time they were described as lunatics and were resident with him at Grove Place. Frederick Duodecimos Dale, a former surgeon had also travelled from Hampshire to Jersey with Pothecary and remained with him until his death in the 1870s. It would appear that as well as attempting to take goods from Grove Place when his lunacy licence was refused, Pothecary also took some of his patients.

Dorothea Dix, the American campaigner for the mentally ill visited Jersey in the 1850s following her trip to Scotland. Dix visited Pothecary's newly arrived lunatics and was very uncomplimentary about his abilities as a carer for the insane. She also visited some of the patients in the hospital, where she found forty lunatics 'in a horrid state, naked, filthy and attended by persons of ill character.' Dix was partly instrumental in persuading the island authorities to fund a new asylum.

With no public facility for lunatics on the island, it was suggested that patients with mental health difficulties could be transferred from the hospital to Pothecary's private asylum. However, following the report of Dorothea Dix, the Lieutenant Governor, Sir Robert Percy Douglas, made the rare decision to exercise his power of veto and successfully blocked this additional delay in building a public asylum when the Home Office and the Commissioners in Lunacy objected that Pothecary was not a fit person to be in charge of lunatics.

Jersey finally gained a public asylum in July 1868 when a new building was opened for use in St Saviour. Twenty-six patients were admitted. At the time of the 1871 census there were fifty-five patients – twenty-nine female and twenty-six male. The medical superintendent was Dr John James Jackson, a native of St Helier, Jersey.

Guernsey
The situation in Guernsey was different to Jersey and a separate asylum had been built by 1852. Prior to this, *The Hospital and Workhouse of the Town and Parish of St Peter Port* had been used for the mentally ill, and in 1851 it was home to nearly 300 assorted paupers, patients and lunatics. As in Jersey, there had been discussions about continuing to use the hospital at St Peter Port as an asylum. However, it was agreed that a separate building was required for those with mental health disorders and the new asylum was erected close to the town hospital. This establishment had room for seventy patients who were cared for by a non-resident medical officer.

The 1861 census reveals that there were thirty-seven patients in the lunatic asylum, which remained attached to the workhouse although the staff for each establishment was different. There were six officers in the asylum, three of whom were related to each other – the master – a former army sergeant, his wife who acted as the mistress of the asylum, and their son. The other staff comprised of a former discharged army pensioner and two house servants. The following decade the number of patients had decreased to twenty-nine, but subsequent years began to show a steady increase.

The presence of the asylum from an early date meant that neither the Lunacy Commissioners nor the Home Office in Westminster were troubled by complaints about the provision of care for the insane in Guernsey until a report on Guernsey lunacy administration was published in the *British Medical Journal* in 1906. As Guernsey fell outside the lunacy legislation for the rest of the British Isles, their laws regarding the incarceration of the insane had not been amended in line with British practice. Whilst in theory this was not a difficulty, the mentally ill of Guernsey were seen to be suffering not only from the dirty conditions within the asylum, but also the consequences of unsatisfactory legislation. There was concern regarding the legalised looseness in the certification of insane persons with nothing in law to prevent family members filling in the necessary medical certificates required for entry into an asylum. By 1906 it had also been brought to light that there were no trained mental or medical nurses in either of the islands' asylums.

Despite Guernsey having led the way with asylum provision in the mid-nineteenth century, providing care for their insane while Jersey deliberated over its position, the roles were reversed fifty years later when Jersey amended its lunacy laws to be in alignment with the rest of the British Isles. Guernsey had not made these changes and its lunacy laws were considered to be inadequate for the requirements of the new century.

The Town Asylum at St Peter Port continued to be attached to the hospital but the area had expanded with industry, including a brewery, which not only made the asylum very dark, but also plagued with rats. It was not until the mid-twentieth century that an up-to-date mental hospital was built for 110 patients in the pleasant area of Le Vauquiedor on Guernsey. It opened in 1940 but was almost immediately requisitioned by the invading Germans who used it for their own military casualties. The mentally ill of Guernsey were returned to their former asylum until the end of the Second World War.

Year	Name and location of establishment
1852	*St Peter Port Town Asylum*, Guernsey.
1868	*Jersey Asylum, St Saviour*, Jersey. Later known as *Jersey Mental Hospital* (1952) and *St Saviour's Hospital*.

Chapter 9

The Isle of Man

The Isle of Man has been a self-governing British Crown dependency in the Irish Sea between Great Britain and Ireland since 1765. It has its own parliament, the High Court of Tynwald, with both upper and lower houses – the Legislative (Lord Lieutenant's) Council and the House of Keys respectively. The head of state is the ruling British monarch, currently Queen Elizabeth, who holds the title of Lord of Mann. The Crown is represented by a Lieutenant Governor on the island. Whilst being separate from the United Kingdom, foreign policy, defence, and good-governance of the dependency are the reserved responsibilities of the Westminster Government in London.

The United Kingdom Government and Crown held great influence in the Isle of Man in the latter half of the nineteenth century, despite legislation having been passed which allowed the island more devolved powers to manage its own affairs.

During his published tour of the Isle of Man in 1794, David Robertson commented that:

The Manks [sic] *are like the Swiss and Highlanders, warmly attached to their native vales and mountains; tenacious of their ancient customs; and jealous of their hereditary rights and privileges. They have however few monuments of public spirit. The House of Keys is a mean building; the public gaol a dungeon; and the principal harbour almost in ruins; while in the whole Island there is no public establishment for sheltering the destitute, protecting the insane, restoring the sick, or supporting the poor. Yet in this country Private charity is liberal.*

During the early part of the nineteenth century there was a lack of provision for the insane on the island. Many individuals with mental health disorders were cared for within the family home – some humanely, others less so. Appropriate provision was clearly needed not just for the insane but also for the poor and sick. Initially it was through charitable bequests that care was provided.

The first official provision for the insane commenced in 1815 when the medieval fortress of Castle Rushen at Castletown was converted for use mainly as a gaol, but also as a place to hold lunatics who were considered dangerous or whose families could no longer control or care for them. As in Wales, several individuals with mental health problems were taken from the Isle of Man to private asylums in England or Scotland. In 1845 the Lieutenant Governor persuaded the Home Office to agree to transfer two criminal lunatics to Haydock Lodge Asylum at Newton-le-Willows between Liverpool and Manchester in northern England. Despite certain controversies surrounding this particular establishment in 1846 that prompted the Welsh counties of Caernarfon and Anglesey to remove their insane from Haydock Lodge, the criminal lunatics of the Isle of Man continued to be sent there. After 1847 however, there was a change of perspective and subsequent cases were sent elsewhere, principally to the Crichton Royal Institution at Dumfries in Scotland.

In February 1849 the Tynwald passed *An Act for the Safe Custody of Insane Persons when Charged with Offences,* which allowed for the safe custody of the insane within Castle Rushen. It allowed 'a person who was supposed to be insane' and who was 'at large' to be brought before the magistrates, and if the person had 'derangement of mind or deficiency of will arising from a defective or vitiated understanding', then they should be sent to Castle Rushen. It stressed that the mentally ill were to be kept separate from the other prisoners. The same Act also made provision for a fund to be set up for the construction of an asylum.

Conditions within Castle Rushen for the insane were far from ideal. In 1851 the British Home Secretary, Sir George Grey (1799–1882), offered to pay the whole of the cost of the maintenance of the criminal lunatics and half the cost of an asylum if the island would pay for the other half. The Lieutenant Governor, the Honourable Charles Hope (1808–93) encouraged the building of an asylum, stating that there were 'a considerable number of lunatics on the Island who ought, both for their own safety and for the safety of others, to be placed in confinement.' A fund was started but an insufficient amount of money was raised and unfortunately it had been deposited in Holmes' Bank (Douglas and Isle of Man Bank) – which collapsed and fell into liquidation on the death of the last surviving partner, James Holmes, a blind 75-year-old, in 1853.

On 1 July 1858 there were eleven lunatics incarcerated in Castle Rushen Gaol. The chaplain of the gaol, Edward Ferrier, MA, and the prison doctor, Thomas Underwood, MD, raised concerns to the Lieutenant Governor and the Tynwald of the appalling conditions these patients were detained in, having committed no crime. They reported that one patient had been admitted there on 22 April 1858, only to commit suicide there on 26 May. They asked for immediate action to be taken to remedy the situation.

The High Court of Tynwald finally passed *The Lunatic Asylum Act* in 1860, providing for the erection and maintenance of an asylum for criminal and pauper lunatics, funded partly out of the general revenue and partly by a lunatic asylum rate. It took a considerable amount of time for the island to raise the necessary funds, and it was not until 1862 that a suitable site was purchased in Strang village in the parish of Bradden, near Douglas.

Case study: Dick Watterson

On 8 February 1864 a letter was published in *The Times* about the prolonged neglect of a lunatic in the Isle of Man. The information had been discovered by William F. Peacock, a Manchester writer who had visited the Isle of Man in the spring of 1863 to write a tourist guide. In July 1863, after rambling 'over every part of the island and thrice round it', he came across an account of a man called Dick Watterson. Peacock managed to find him in the village of Ballakillowey. Watterson was 34-years-old but for the previous seventeen years had been bricked up, alive and alone. The 1861 census indicates that he had been insane since the age of 18 but was resident with his widowed mother Ann, who farmed fourteen acres. Peacock described the conditions he was living in by writing:

The walls of his filthy cow-house are damp and unsightly; a morsel of foul straw varies the squalid monotony of the cold clay floor; and Dick Watterson is naked save a loose sack which now and then he throws on his shivering shoulders. I forbear to speak of the ordure of the place, of the countless vermin which inhabit

*his (otherwise fair and soft) skin, and of other even more
disgusting matters.*

In October 1863, Peacock brought the case to the attention of the
Lieutenant Governor who wrote back to him 'most feelingly', though
Watterson was still in his cow shed in January 1864.

In 1864, the Tynwald Court appointed a managing committee of at least
five members and a rate was set for the new asylum. John Henry Christian
was appointed architect. The new Isle of Man Lunatic Asylum at
Ballamona, was opened on 2 June 1868 at a total cost of £15,149. Seventy-
six patients were admitted on opening including Richard Watterson. Within
the first thirty years of its existence the patient population doubled and
extensions were added to the asylum to accommodate the increase. The
asylum was renamed Isle of Man Mental Hospital in 1934, then Ballamona
Hospital in 1955. With the shift to 'care in the community' in the 1980s,
Ballamona Hospital closed and the buildings were finally demolished in
1998 to make way for a new hospital.

In 1870, Rev James Elkey Pattison, Curate of Lezayre, published the
following rhyme about the asylum in his work *Manxiana: Rhymes and
Legends.*

THE ASYLUM
'Tis built, and not too soon, I think,
For many hundred years o'er all the Isle,
In towns and villages along the shore,
On the wide Curragh, up among the hills,
Along the plains, and o'er the lonely moors,
High up by the valley of the Sulby stream,
Amongst the giant boulders on the base
Of Snaefell's rugged height— there wandered free
The Tom o'Bedlams of our Mona's isle;
The Peter Greys, and Bettys of the Drun,
Were everywhere — outraging decency,
In rags that made the nakedness more sad
Than Indian Fakeer of the Himalaya hills.
Now the Asylum's built, a noble pile,
A home for all — well worthy of the Isle.

Chapter 10

Life in the Asylum

In nineteenth century Britain and Ireland, asylums became the permanent home for many people who were considered mentally ill. Patients who had been incarcerated in the most basic and primitive form of establishment at the beginning of the century would have experienced a huge change in the level of both comfort and care as conditions improved thanks to new legislation. For many working class people, despite the continued stigma of asylums, there was a huge difference in terms of food and accommodation and as a result, many patients were glad to be away from workhouse or gaol provision.

Accommodation
Nineteenth century asylums were built with the comfort and safety of patients in mind. Those that were constructed following Dr William A.F. Browne's utopian vision of therapeutic palaces and Dr John Conolly's recommendations regarding *The Construction and Government of Lunatic Asylums* were deemed more comfortable than those in existence at the beginning of the century. New buildings and grounds were constructed with a clear aim and purpose – the therapeutic care of patients in a secure and protected environment and with the strict segregation of men and women. The choice of location for new asylums was an important consideration and most were built at a distance from towns with a pleasant aspect and a good supply of clean fresh water. Good railway links were important for the transportation of patients and some asylums had their own railway station.

The architecture of asylums was of huge importance for financial, therapeutic and safety reasons. As new buildings were designed, particular attention was paid to maximum security, ventilation and efficient drainage.

In the first half of the nineteenth century, new county or district asylums were designed by the County Architect, generally in consultation with the Lunacy Commissioners and medical superintendents. However, such was the demand for new asylum buildings following improved legislation in the latter part of the century that some architects began to specialise in their design and construction. George Thomas Hine (1842–1916) was an English architect who won many competitions with his designs and was responsible for the construction of a large number of asylums during the nineteenth century, including four for London County Council. Another architect who specialised in the planning of asylums, prisons and hospitals was Robert J. Griffiths, Architect and County Surveyor for the County of Staffordshire (d. 1888 at Highfield Grove, Stafford). Griffiths was the architect responsible for the design and supervision of Cheshire's second county asylum, Parkside in Macclesfield, which opened in May 1871. The style he chose for Parkside was Italianate in the 'Rundbogenstil' or 'rounded arch style'. It was fitted-out using the best quality materials, including mahogany lavatory seats, hot running water and a maple dance floor. The level of luxury it provided must have been extreme for many of its inhabitants and there remains no doubt that Dr W.A.F. Browne would have approved of the large airy rooms, quality fittings and extensive grounds.

Due to the large number of staff required for the maintenance and running of an asylum, as well as the increasing number of patients requiring asylum care, asylums resembled self-contained stately homes with their own farms, lodge keepers and ornamental gardens. The grounds were designed by landscape gardeners and special attention was given to bowling greens, croquet lawns and cricket pitches. Many asylums had their own cricket and football teams made up of a combination of male attendants and patients. There were 'airing courts' and walled gardens with shelters where patients could safely exercise in the fresh air. Some asylums had drinking fountains in the airing courts but, for safety reasons, patient access to water was restricted and lakes were never designed as an external architectural feature. At Denbigh Asylum in North Wales, a reservoir was constructed in the 1870s to conserve water for patient use, but it was guarded by a 10 ft high fence to deter those of a suicidal inclination. Later the same decade fire hydrants were connected to the town's water supply in case of fire.

Many larger asylums had their own fire brigade and fire engine, which would have been manned by the male attendants assisted when possible by the male patients. The third Surrey County Pauper Lunatic Asylum opened in December 1883 in Coulsdon, Surrey had its own fire station as the closest one at Purley, Surrey was considered too far away from such a large establishment. Some asylums were not so forward thinking however, and the fire at Colney Hatch Asylum in 1903 claimed many lives despite the asylum having its own fire brigade, which proved ineffective against the flames.

Internally, asylums were split into two halves: one for male patients and the other for females. As halves, they generally mirrored each other and both contained a variety of wards for different classes of patient. Patients were regularly required to sleep in dormitories built to accommodate up to fifty people and there was only a minimal level of privacy when it came to washing and dressing. The larger dormitories were assigned to those considered to be 'moderately tranquil' and smaller rooms were available for those considered to be 'refractory'. In some asylums with a large number of epileptic patients there was a separate dormitory or wing for their care. Single rooms were also available, but they were used for disturbed patients and those thought to be unwell. Many epileptic patients were given single rooms. Peep holes in the doors enabled asylum staff to check on patients at intervals during the night without disturbing them.

There were allocated areas of seclusion for patients in terms of both padded and secluded rooms. Following John Conolly's recommendations that restraint be abolished, most forms of mechanical restraint such as coercion chairs, leg locks and other types of ironmongery ceased to be used by the mid-nineteenth century. Linen jackets with buttons down the back and long sleeves with tapes on the ends remained for the most difficult patients as straight jackets or straight waistcoats. Gloves without fingers, fastened at the wrist with buttons or locks were also used to prevent self-injury, to stop the patients removing dressings from wounds, to ensure they could not induce vomiting by putting their fingers down their throats, and to prevent them from tearing their bedding or clothing into strips with which to hang themselves. However, restraint was only used as a last resort and each one had to be sanctioned and witnessed by the medical superintendent and recorded in a Register of Restraints that could be inspected by the Lunacy Commissioners.

As in any institution, the patients lived and worked by the clock – an existence which many would have been accustomed to in their experiences in workhouses or poorhouses, but for others it was an alien concept which heightened their awareness of incarceration. For many patients the asylum routine was a comfort, but for others it was stifling and exacerbated their mental condition. The longer a patient remained in the asylum, the more institutionalised they became – accepting the drudging routine of institutionalised life as a normality – many became docile and accepted their fate.

Most asylums woke their patients at 6 am in the summer and 7 am in the winter. Men who were able to work were taken out to the farm or quarry or employed outdoors and women spent time sewing, embroidering, or knitting while the dormitories and wards were cleaned before breakfast at 8 am. The patients' day was interspersed with regular meal intervals and in the majority of asylums, men and women ate in the same room albeit at different tables or at different times.

Parkside Asylum in Cheshire had its own ballroom, which was also used as a theatre and for concerts – it had space for a sixteen-piece orchestra and was decorated with potted plants. Other parts of the asylum were similarly decorated with lace curtains, pictures and pretty stencils on the walls. The purpose was to ensure the asylum was as pleasant and cheerful as possible to aid the psychological treatment of the patients and also to deter those with destructive tendencies and help restrain their behaviour.

Food

The food allowance per patient was measured by weight depending on their gender. At Parkside Asylum in Cheshire in 1888, breakfast consisted of six ounces of bread, half an ounce of butter and a pint of coffee or cocoa for men and an ounce less of bread for women. Dinner varied each day, with meat served four times a week and fish every Friday. Additional provisions were given to malnourished paupers and those in the infirmary were provided with supplements on the advice of the medical staff. The dining tables were set in rows each with a tablecloth that was renewed twice a week.

The food allowance at Denbigh Asylum was not as generous as Parkside but was monitored by the visiting commissioners and was generally deemed to be of good quality. Men were allocated seven ounces of meat and women six ounces three days a week with an allocation of three ounces of Australian meat twice a week and suet pudding once a week. Male pauper patients were given an allowance of beer until 1879 when this was discontinued except during harvest time and seasonal activities such as Christmas.

Clothing
At the beginning of the nineteenth century many asylum patients were ill-clad and provided with only the basic of coverings for warmth. Following the 1808 County Asylums Act few counties built asylums to house their insane and therefore acquiring the necessary funds to clothe them was not a high priority.

When Dr John Conolly was medical superintendent at Hanwell during the 1840s, he recommended that patients in asylums should be adequately clothed to maintain their physical and mental wellbeing. In his opinion the mode of dress chosen by a lunatic was an indication of their mental state and it was the responsibility of asylum staff to ensure that their clothing was both warm and functional.

The clothing of patients in an asylum of any description merits very careful attention, both as one of the means of preserving health, and as one of the things re-acting on the mind. Among the most constant indications of insanity are to be observed negligence or peculiarity as to dress; and many patients seem to lose the power of regulating it according to the seasons, or the weather, or the customs of society. As regards the clothing of the pauper lunatic in a county asylum, it is especially desirable that it should be warm, both in the winter and in the changeable weather of the autumn and spring, and cool and unirritating in the summer. The vernal excitement so distinctly visible in the wards, seems to suggest particular attention to the clothing at the season when the temperature becomes rather suddenly elevated, after the severities of the winter and early spring. The irritability of some of the patients, and the coldness and increased feebleness of others, show the importance of warm winter clothing for patients suffering from various forms of nervous disturbance, many of which seem to interfere with the function of animal heat. Many of the insane, also, are predisposed to pulmonary consumption, and a flannel waistcoat or drawers are indispensable to them, as well as to those who become depressed and inactive in severe weather.

Warm worsted stockings, and cloth boots or shoes, kept in good repair, are very essential to some of them. The slovenly character given to most of the imbecile and maniacal patients by the falling down of their stockings over their ankles, might be avoided, I imagine, by the structure of the upper part of the stocking being assimilated to that of children's half-stockings, which are easily kept up; or an elastic band at the top of the stocking might be convenient. Garters are generally lost or misapplied, and strings are inconvenient or useless. In these matters, the physician should be aided by female sub-officers, willing to learn and ready to assist. Boots made of cloth are much worn at Hanwell, and seem very useful; if necessary, they are fastened on by a small lock, instead of a button. Stout linen is the material used both for men's shirts and women's under garments at Hanwell. Some of the female patients, unaccustomed to course apparel, complain of the skin being irritated by the linen, and calico is occasionally substituted for it. The men have clean shirts twice a week, and the attendants and officers should not permit them to be worn without buttons. A great number of the patients will keep themselves clean and neat if allowed to do so.

Not every asylum complied with a uniform mode of dress although many did provide 'wearing apparel' for the patients, which distinguished them from the staff in the asylum. Many patients had their own clothes removed for hygiene reasons but in some cases individuals retained their clothing, which provided them with a degree of normality in a situation far from their choosing.

In Parkside Asylum in Macclesfield, Cheshire, the patients did not wear clothes that could be described as a uniform. Those who did not have sufficient clothing of their own were provided with items by the asylum. The men wore cloth, moleskin or corduroy trousers and had a change of linen twice a week. Women had gowns of cotton, linsey or wool depending on the season. Plaid shawls were common but 'dirty' patients had strong, linen jackets, allowing skirts to be removed for reasons of cleanliness without completely undressing the patient.

The attendants and nurses at Parkside did not wear uniform until the beginning of the twentieth century – prior to this they wore the 'ordinary attire of everyday life' to make the asylum feel less like an institution.

At the Royal Edinburgh Asylum in 1855 the men were allowed flannel waistcoats and drawers, which were changed once a fortnight, and they had a clean shirt once a week. A similar method of dress was also issued at Murray's Asylum, Perth in the same year but shirts were changed twice a week.

Patients at Denbigh Asylum wore hospital clothing and most were only issued with one set of clothes until Sunday Uniforms were issued in 1876 which gave the patients a lot of pleasure.

Canvas dresses, fastened by locks, were occasionally placed on destructive and paralytic patients. Thick cloth clothing that was difficult to tear into strips was regularly provided to patients of a suicidal nature and their shoes and boots were also closed with a lock instead of bootlaces.

Hygiene

Promoting good hygiene was a constant battle for asylum staff who dealt with a large number of 'dirty' or incontinent patients on a daily basis. Whilst many of the newer asylums were built with internal bathrooms and hot running water near to dormitories, this was not the case in every county. Bathing was a supervised communal activity with baths generally positioned in the centre of the room so that attendants could gather around bathers for their safety. Whilst a certain amount of privacy was provided during the use of lavatories, the doors would have no bolts and were open at the top and bottom so that attendants could check on patient's welfare while they were inside.

Turkish baths were considered to have both a cleansing and therapeutic effect in cases of insanity and were also recognised as beneficial in cases of consumption and rheumatism. The asylum in Cork had a Turkish bath attached to the institution. The asylum visitors at Denbigh travelled to the asylums at both Cork and Limerick in 1870 to learn more about the benefits and were impressed enough to have them built for Denbigh.

Unfortunately, in Cork in 1889, part of the bath became defective and nearly caused the death of fifty-six patients who inhaled poisonous gas and smoke which crept through the crevices of the bath when they entered the room. It was only due to the quick intervention of medical officers that fatalities were prevented.

Patient employment

Employment was considered an important part of moral therapy and men were encouraged to continue with the trade they were trained for, or in the labouring tasks they had before admission, whether as agricultural or general labourers. Women were similarly employed within the laundry and sewing room and also assisted with the general housekeeping of the asylum, scrubbing floors and polishing furniture. Employing patients in this way was considered to be making them useful and less anxious about their incarceration, and to build up their self-esteem as useful, valuable members of the community. Many patient case notes reflect the calming influence of domestic tasks.

Making, repairing, and cleaning clothes was a huge job within the asylum and provided a major source of employment for female patients and staff. In the industrial north-west of England and the Border counties of Scotland, many patients had previously been employed in the textile industry and therefore had specialist skills when it came to working with

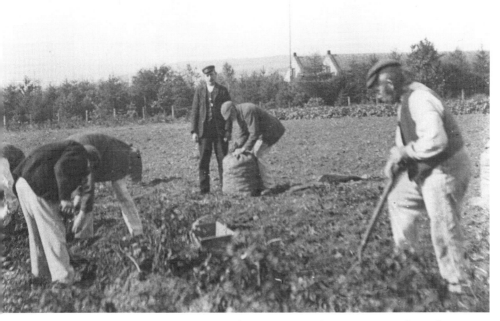

Potato gathering on the farm at Dundee Lunatic Asylum. Courtesy of Dundee University Archive Services.

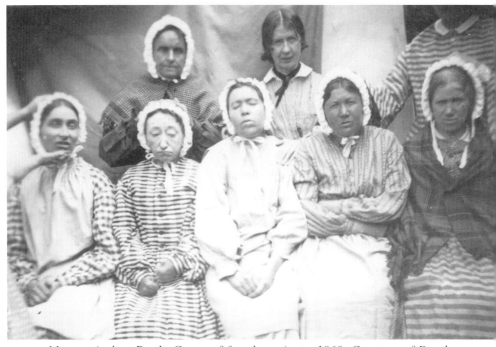

Murray Asylum Perth. Group of female patients, 1860. Courtesy of Dundee University Archive Services.

Murray Asylum Perth. Group of male patients, 1860. Courtesy of Dundee University Archive Services.

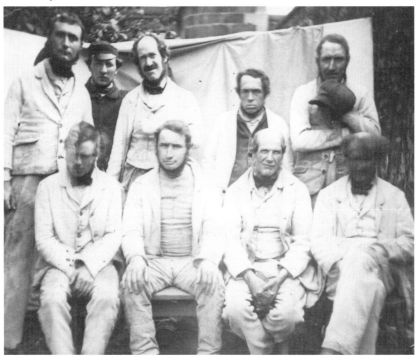

cloth. Even in areas that were considered more rural such as remote parts of Wales, Scotland and Ireland, people had far more skills when it came to dressmaking and tailoring than would be seen today. These skills were an important way of keeping the mentally ill occupied, whilst ensuring that the patients always had adequate clothing.

Asylums employed skilled tradesmen such as shoemakers, blacksmiths and engineers and the patients worked alongside these people using the skills they already had, but also acquiring new ones to aid in the running of the institution. The majority of asylums had a farm, land and market garden, which were used to provide food for the patients and staff. The male patients in particular were encouraged to help with the farm labour and gardening. Those unsuited to outdoor work were often requested to repair bedding and clean hair and flock mattresses.

At the Surrey County Lunatic Asylum at Brookwood patients and attendants were reported to work together in such harmony and companionship that it was often difficult to differentiate between them. Outdoor labour and works carried on within the asylum were arranged to provide varied sources of interest and promote positive remedial treatment.

Leisure activities
Recreation was considered an important part of recovery and rehabilitation and asylums provided many activities for the benefit of patients. Asylum staff were expected to participate and encourage patients to avail themselves of the opportunities provided for them. Music, dancing, libraries and sport were just some of the activities available to those willing to participate.

Music and theatre
At the Crichton Royal Institution in Dumfries, Scotland, Dr W.A.F. Browne (1805–85) introduced a variety of activities 'to sweeten confinement, and to promote the cheerfulness of minds' of the patients as early as 1840. One of these was music. Browne considered music to be a means of bringing the asylum community together. A variety of instruments were played by patients in the wards, at concerts, and at asylum theatricals, and also by asylum staff. In 1840, Glasgow Royal Asylum paid for a music teacher to give music lessons twice a week. As a result, patients learned new skills and gained confidence.

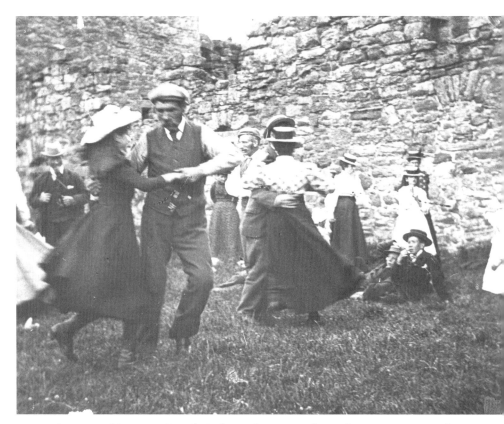

Dancing, Montrose Royal Asylum. Courtesy of Dundee University Archive Services.

Together with concerts, lectures and dances, there were 'magical lantern' shows and theatrical performances. In 1843 Browne staged a successful farce *Raising the Wind* at the Crichton Institute which featured both staff and patients in the cast. It was well received and enthusiastically reviewed in the *Dumfries Herald.*

At Hanwell Asylum one of the favoured indoor recreations for the patients during the winter days and evenings was music. In the 1840s the asylum purchased three pianos, flutes, clarinets, and violins for patients who could play. Some of the attendants were good musicians and a small band was formed to provide entertainment at winter evening parties.

Worcester City and County Lunatic Asylum employed Edward Elgar (1857–1934) one day a week in the asylum band. In 1879, at the age of 22, he was appointed asylum bandmaster. His duties were to train and conduct the band, which comprised solely of asylum attendants. He was expected to have a practical knowledge of the flute, oboe, clarinet, euphonium and all string instruments and was paid £32 per annum. In addition he was paid 5s for each polka and quadrille he composed for the band to play.

Adverts for asylum attendants regularly specified that they sought individuals who could play musical instruments. At Parkside Asylum in Cheshire in the 1890s, adverts were placed for attendants who could play the euphonium, and a first violinist at a salary of £30 per annum with uniform, board, lodging and laundry included.

Asylum dances and balls
An asylum ball afforded much amusement – not only for the patients but also for groups of local dignitaries invited to attend. On these occasions music was often provided by the asylum band, which would regularly comprise both attendants and patients, or the asylum would hire a troop of musicians for the evening's entertainment. The ballroom was brightly decorated and fancy dress was a regular favourite. Patients were not generally permitted to spend the entire evening among the guests and were often put to bed by the attendants at about 10pm. Charles Maurice Davies (1828–1910), was an Anglican clergyman, a prolific author and a spiritualist who wrote *Mystic London* in which he recounted his experiences as a member of 'Herr Gustav Küster's corps of fiddlers' when they played at an asylum ball at Hanwell Asylum in 1875.

High jinks commenced at the early hour of six; and long before that time we had deposited our instruments in the Bazaar, as the ball-room is somewhat incongruously called, and were threading the Daedalean mazes of the wards. Life in the wards struck me as being very like living in a passage; but when that preliminary objection was got over, the long corridors looked comfortable enough. They were painted in bright warm colours, and a correspondingly genial temperature was secured by hot-water pipes running the entire length. Comfortable rooms opened out from the wards at frequent intervals, and there was every form of amusement to beguile the otherwise irksome leisure of those temporary recluses. Most of my hermits were smoking – I mean on the male side – many were reading; one had a fiddle, and scraped acquaintance immediately with him; whilst another was seated at the door of his snug little bedroom, getting up cadenzas on the flute. He was an old trombone-player in one of the household regiments, an inmate of Hanwell for thirty years, and a fellow bandsman with myself for the evening. He looked, I thought, quite as sane as myself, and played magnificently; but I was informed by the possibly prejudiced officials that he had his occasional weaknesses. A second member of Herr Kuster's band whom I found in durance was a clarionet [sic] player formerly in the band of the Second Life Guards; and this poor fellow, who was an excellent musician too, felt his position acutely. He apologized sotto voce for sitting down with me in corduroys, as well as for being an 'imbecile'. He did not seem to question the justice of the verdict against him, and had not become acclimatized to the atmosphere like the old trombone-player.

That New Year's night – for January was very young – the wards, especially on the women's side, were gaily decorated with paper flowers, and all looked as cheerful and happy as though no shadow ever fell across the threshold; but, alas, there were every now and then padded rooms opening out of the passage; and as this was not a refractory ward, I asked the meaning of the arrangement, which I had fancied was an obsolete one. I was told they were for epileptic patients. In virtue of his official position as bandmaster, Herr Kuster had a key; and, after walking serenely into a passage precisely like the rest, informed me, with the utmost coolness, that I was in the refractory ward. I looked around for the stalwart attendant, who is generally to be seen on duty, and to my dismay found he was quite at the other end of an exceedingly long corridor. I do not know that I am particularly nervous; but I candidly confess to an anxiety to get near that worthy official. We were only three outsiders, and the company looked mischievous. One gentleman was walking violently up and down, turning up his coat-sleeves, as though bent on our instant demolition. Another, an old grey-bearded man, came up, and fiercely demanded if I were a Freemason. I was afraid he might resent my saying I was not, when it happily occurred to me that the third in our party, an amateur contra-bassist, was of the craft. I told our old friend so. He demanded the sign, was satisfied, and, in the twinkling of an eye, our double-bass friend was struggling in his fraternal embrace. The warder, mistaking the character of the hug, hastened to the rescue, and I was at ease.

We then passed to the ball-room, where my musical friends were beginning to 'tune up,' and waiting for their conductor. The large room was gaily decorated, and filled with some three or four hundred patients, arranged Spurgeon-wise: the ladies on one side, and the gentlemen on the other. There was a somewhat rakish air about the gathering, due to the fact of the male portion not being in full dress, but arrayed in free-and-easy costume of corduroys and felt boots. The frequent warders in their dark blue uniforms lent quite a military air to the scene; and on the ladies' side the costumes were more picturesque; some little latitude was given to feminine taste, and the result was that a large portion of the patients were gorgeous in pink gowns. One old lady, who claimed to be a scion of royalty, had a resplendent mob-cap; but the belles of the ball-room were decidedly to be found among the female attendants, who were bright, fresh-looking young women, in a neat, black uniform, with perky little caps, and bunches of keys hanging at their side like the rosary of a soeur de charité, or the chatelaines with which young ladies love to adorn themselves at present. Files of patients kept streaming into the already crowded room, and one gentleman, reversing the order assigned to him by nature, walked gravely in on the palms of his hands, with his legs elevated in air. He had been a clown at a theatre, and still retained some of the proclivities of the boards. A wizen-faced man, who seemed to have no name beyond the conventional one of 'Billy', strutted in with huge paper collars, like the corner mail in a nigger troupe, and a tin decoration on his breast the size of a cheeseplate. He was insensible to the charms of Terpsichore, except in the shape of an occasional pas seul, and laboured under the idea that his mission was to conduct the band, which he occasionally did, to the discomfiture of Herr Kuster, and the total destruction of gravity on the part of the executants, so that Billy had to be displaced. It was quite curious to notice the effect of the music on some of the quieter patients. One or two, whose countenances really seemed to justify their incarceration, absolutely hugged the foot of my music-stand, and would not allow me to hold my instrument for a moment when I was not playing on it, so anxious were they to express their admiration of me as an artist. 'I used to play that instrument afore I come here', said a patient, with a squeaky voice, who for eleven years has laboured under the idea that his mother is coming to see him on the morrow; indeed, most of the little group around the platform looked upon their temporary sojourn at Hanwell as the only impediment to a bright career in the musical world.

Another hour, rapidly passed in the liberal hospitality of this great institution, and silence had fallen on its congregated thousands. It is a small town in itself, and to a large extent self-dependent and self-governed. It bakes and brews, and makes its gas; and there is no need of a Licensing Bill to keep its inhabitants sober and steady. The method of doing that has been discovered in nature's own law of kindness. Instead of being chained and treated as wild beasts, the lunatics are treated as unfortunate men and women, and every effort is made to ameliorate, both physically and morally, their sad condition. Hence the bright wards, the buxom attendants, the frequent jinks. Even the chapel-service has been brightened up for their behoof.

This was what I saw by entering as an amateur fiddler Herr Kuster's band at Hanwell Asylum; and as I ran to catch the last up-train – which I did as the saying is by the skin of my teeth – I felt that I was a wiser, though it may be a sadder man, for my evening's experiences at the Lunatic Ball.

At the New Year's Eve ball at Denbigh in 1876 dancing began at 7pm and the patients enjoyed the festivities and were allowed to dance until 9pm when they were served hot broth, plum pudding and coffee. Visitors to the ball remained until after midnight when the National Anthem was played. To make up for their early departure from the festivities, the attendants had a separate event a week later.

In 1870 the Christmas festivities at Chester Lunatic Asylum in Cheshire included a dance of Polkas, Galops and Quadrilles and the musical delights of visits from dramatic and choral societies. A special attraction: *Dissolving views run by elaborate machinery and illuminated by limelight* was the highlight of the Christmas period and an early form of cinema.

At the Surrey County Lunatic Asylum at Brookwood a fancy dress ball was an annual occurrence. The recreation hall was decorated with

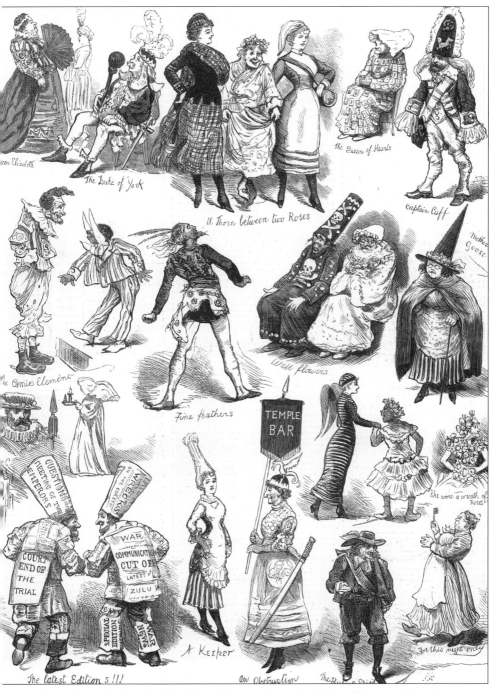

Fancy Dress Ball at the Brookwood Surrey Lunatic Asylum. Illustrated London News, 1881.

exotic plants, flags, wreaths, statuettes, mirrors and Chinese lanterns. Music was provided by the asylum band and patients and staff wore a costume. At the ball in 1881 the medical superintendent Dr Thomas Nadauld Brushfield (1828–1910) dressed as a Hunchback called 'The Ruling Spirit', while his assistants, Dr Barton and Dr Moody respectively took on the guise of a Japanese warrior and the Duke of Marlborough.

At the Royal Edinburgh Asylum there was a weekly ball and concert, which was much looked forward to by the patients. The ball room was able to host up to 300 people who ate currant buns and drank whisky punch whilst enjoying country dances, singing and dramatic recitations performed by patients, staff and visitors.

Libraries

By the mid-nineteenth century most asylums provided reading material for their patients. Many asylums had libraries and provided daily and weekly newspapers, magazines, illustrated periodicals and general literature including the Bible. Reading was considered as a means of uplifting and improving the mind and also a way of helping to educate asylum patients.

Lincoln Asylum had an impressive library of books on natural history as early as 1834. Other asylums had equally large libraries and patients were noted to gain great pleasure from having books to read. Books were generally selected by the chaplain and would have been chosen with care and the contents examined for the likely influence they would have had on the reader.

Dr William Mackinnon, physician superintendent of the Royal Edinburgh Asylum at Morningside between 1839–46, installed a printing press and encouraged the publication of the hospital magazine, *The Morningside Mirror.* This magazine published by both patients and staff ran from 1845 until 1974. As the title suggests, the magazine allowed patients to reflect on their lives and thoughts whilst in the asylum. In 1852 a patient named Alexis, a regular contributor to the magazine, wrote:

How changed is the treatment of the insane in my recollection! With that sedulous attention and gentleness, contrasted with the cruel, because ignorant, discipline of former days, are they cared for! Coercion and restraint have been superseded by mercy and regulated liberty.

Patients were encouraged to participate in amusements to relieve the monotony of institutional life and to interact with one another.

Church services
Most asylums also had their own church or chapel and quite often a cemetery although this was not the case in every county. Religious instruction and observance was seen as a significant part of moral therapy, giving support and comfort to patients. In most asylums church services were provided on a weekly basis, sometimes more frequently, but attendance was not compulsory and male and female patients were segregated for the duration of the service. The Glasgow Royal Asylum annual report of 1821 made recommendations for a proposed chapel:

> *The means of separating the males from the females, so that they shall not be able to see each other, while they may have it in the power to see the clergyman; and also the means of separating the patients of the higher ranks from their inferiors.*

Having a separate building of a chapel or church was important, rather than providing religious services within the main asylum in one of the

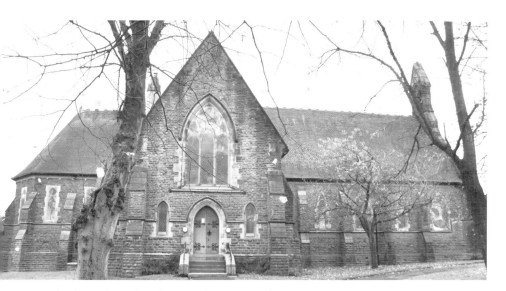

Parkside Asylum Church. © Kathryn Burtinshaw.

halls or dining areas. The physical act of 'going to church' on a Sunday was a weekly event in itself which most inmates had been accustomed to prior to admission. Permitting patients to follow a lifestyle as close as possible to their pre-asylum status was beneficial.

The church built for the Glamorgan County Lunatic Asylum was described as 'a neat little Gothic structure' and could seat 250 patients. This church matched in many ways the architecture of the asylum. The church at Parkside looked very different from the asylum buildings, and was a later addition to the institution. Due to the large number of epileptic patients at Parkside, the rear pews of the church were wider in case of seizures during the service.

Outdoor activities

Exercise was considered an important part of moral treatment and patients took frequent walks in the airing courts and the grounds of the asylum. On occasion they were taken further afield into the wider community accompanied by asylum staff. At Denbigh Asylum, patients who did not work were sent out into the airing courts for much of the day. Rainy days were considered difficult and awnings and corrugated iron coverings were erected so that patients were not 'deprived' of the fresh outdoors.

Some medical superintendents were criticised for allowing patients outside the walls of the asylum. Thomas Steele Sheldon (1856–1952), medical superintendent at Parkside Asylum, encouraged trips and walking parties and responded to criticism with – 'It is a pleasure to be able to record the humanity shown in our walking parties by farmers, cottagers and – shopkeepers.' His sensitivity may in part be explained due to the mental incapacity of his father Thomas George Sheldon who had been admitted to and died in a private asylum called The Brook Villa, Private Institution for the Care of Patients of Unsound Mind, in West Derby, Liverpool in 1903. Without doubt, this would have given Sheldon a greater personal understanding of the impact of mental instability on a family. Thomas Steele Sheldon was frequently known to express the opinion 'we must try and make this place more like a hospital and less a place of restraint, and treat the patients as individuals not as cases.'

Some asylums organised annual picnics to provide the patients with a change of scene, fresh air and the opportunity to escape the routine of the asylum. The *Morningside Mirror* of 15 August 1884 described the enjoyment of both staff and patients of the Edinburgh Royal Asylum following their annual picnic to the Braid Hills.

The great annual picnic of the West House inmates to the Braid Hills came off on Thursday, 31 July. About 11 A.M. some 500 of the male and female inmates were assembled on the lawn in front of West House, and on the signal being given, the procession moved off in fine order, headed by two pipers, and carrying gay flags and banners at intervals. Issuing by the east gate, they turned up the hill road to the south-east, and soon reached the Braid Hills field. Here they rested after their march, and partook of a luncheon of bread and biscuits with cheese and beer and lemonade in large quantities. They now dispersed in parties to climb about the hills, and they so spent a long time in their happy rambles. The early part of the day was rather foggy, but it soon cleared up, and the sun shone out beautifully in the afternoon and evening. Dinner was taken between two and three, and the large supply of beefsteak pies and rhubarb and gooseberry tarts disappeared very rapidly. After a little rest dancing was begun and kept up with much spirit till far on in the evening, to the lively music of Mr Black's band. The other and usual sports were also engaged in, such as running, jumping, carrying or 'lifting' the Doctors and officials, amid much fun and laughter, and ineffectual struggles on the part of those who were so highly honoured and shouldered. About 7 P.M. the great multitude began their march homewards, and when all had arrived in front of the West House, an ample tea, with bread and jam, was served to everyone. After some more frolics and fun, the large assemblage broke up and retired, all very much wearied, yet delighted with their grand yearly picnic on the Braids, and, no doubt, longing for next year's holiday of the same kind.

Sport

Sporting activities, particularly for the male patients were very much favoured and encouraged. Most asylums had their own football and cricket teams comprising both attendants and patients. At the Edinburgh Royal Asylum the first physician superintendent, Dr William Mackinnon, had a curling pond constructed and encouraged the patients to participate in competitions with other curling clubs.

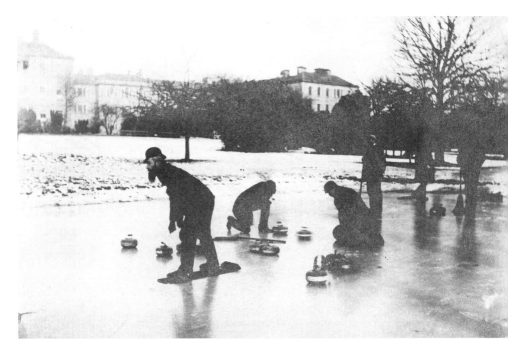

Curling at Royal Edinburgh Asylum. Courtesy of Lothian Health Services Archive.

At Denbigh Asylum special attention was paid to improve the lack of purposeful outdoor activities. An area of ground was allotted and levelled to form a bowling green, and quoiting and skittle grounds were also laid out. The labour costs for these improvements were minimal as the male patients provided the majority of the work.

Many asylums also encouraged cricket matches during the summer months; at Broadmoor in 1881, however, this nearly led to the escape of two of the patients, John Biggs and Joseph Waller, both of whom had been charged with murder but acquitted on grounds of insanity. During the game the ball was hit to the boundary of the field and both Biggs and Waller went in hot pursuit. No particular notice was taken of this, the warders imagining that the fieldsmen were simply trying to retrieve the ball. However, noticing that they passed the spot where the ball bounded, and observing that they went ahead at a great pace, two of the warders went in pursuit and caught the patients in the woods outside the asylum grounds.

John Biggs was an 18-year-old millwright who had cut the throat of his sweetheart, Mary Ann Bromwich, with a razor in Leicester in 1879.

Joseph Waller was a 24-year-old labourer convicted of the double murder of his former employers Edward and Elizabeth Ellis in Chislehurst, Kent on 31 October 1880. Both Biggs and Waller had committed brutal murders but an examination of both declared them to be insane and they were sent to Broadmoor. More information about these two men is contained within Chapter 12, *The Criminal Lunatic*.

Most asylums had their own cricket and football pitches and some had tennis courts. Fixtures were set up for matches against local school and community teams. However, for administrative and security reasons, the games were always played within asylum grounds. There were also inter-asylum fixtures where the team from one asylum would play against that of another. There are accounts of cricket matches in the 1880s between the Royal Edinburgh Asylum and the Fife and Kinross District Asylum at Springfield, near Cupar. The Edinburgh team travelled by train to Leith, took a steamer across the Forth estuary to Burntisland, then another train to Cupar, and finally horse-drawn carriages to Springfield. They were well catered for by the medical superintendent, Dr Adam Turnbull, and stayed overnight in Fife after the match before returning to Edinburgh the following day.

Sporting activities were, however, very much a male preserve. Women were not encouraged to participate in team games but were instead taken for long walks or provided with sewing or knitting to keep them occupied. On occasions, being confined purposelessly for lengthy periods in the airing courts had a negative impact on their mental health and did more harm than good.

Visitors

Visits from family and friends were regulated and, for many pauper patients, there would have been no hope of receiving visitors due to the long distances they would have to travel. Similarly letters from patients were censored by the medical superintendent – who read all communications in case they contained inaccurate or misleading information. Letters to the Lunacy Commissioners were exempt from this, allowing patients to make complaints about their treatment if they wished. Similarly, patients were allowed to speak to the Lunacy Commissioners when visits to the asylum took place.

Visits from family and friends were regularly fraught with anxiety for both the patient and those visiting them. There was regularly a deep resentment and blame by patients who believed their relatives were responsible for having placed them in the asylum, generally without due cause. Others were ashamed to be seen dressed in asylum clothes and locked away for reasons of insanity. Patients were able to receive letters from family and friends but this was not always conducive to their mental health.

Case study: Mary Lowe
Mary Barker Lowe was admitted to Parkside from her home on 20 September 1897 with mania and epilepsy. She wrote numerous letters complaining about her surroundings and was eventually discharged into the care of her friends on 25 March 1898.

Case study: Mary Dickenson
Mary Dickenson, an epileptic patient, was admitted to Parkside from Altrincham Workhouse in Knutsford, Cheshire where she had been resident for twelve months. As her seizures increased in number, so did her complaints, and she frequently requested that her medication should be changed. Mary accused the asylum nurses of ill treatment and of causing her bruises, but no evidence could be found by the medical officers to back up her claims.

Mentally she was querulous, always asking to go home – but her nearest relatives declined to admit her on account of the great trouble she had given them in the past. Her relatives repeatedly replied to her letters stating that they did not want anything to do with her, which made Mary very perturbed and determined to go home to sort things out. Each time she became agitated her seizures and restlessness increased and she became a very unsettled patient.

Case study: Jane McLoughlin
Jane McLoughlin was initially admitted to Parkside on 15 August 1885 and diagnosed with mania. The medical officer wrote a detailed physical and mental report on her condition and observed that she was 'hardworking with brutal husband'. Her husband John was also described 'as not a sober man'. There is no suggestion however, that he was accountable for his wife's condition or incapable of caring for their children.

Jane was described as 'unmanageable' in the early stages of her admission to Parkside. She crawled on the floor on her hands and knees and wandered around in a semi-naked state as if she was looking for someone. Within a couple of weeks she seemed more content, began to smile and spoke more rationally. However, she had a great objection to seeing her husband. In November 1885 following one month's trial, she was discharged and deemed recovered.

Her second admission to Parkside occurred six years later in 1891 and her mental and physical condition had deteriorated dramatically. Described as 'moribund and exhausted', she needed support from her two companions. She was diagnosed with epileptic mania; frequent childbearing was provided as a reason for her condition. The case notes record that she had had thirteen children, the youngest of whom had been born three years earlier. Jane died in an exhausted state three days after admittance and before the Medical Superintendent had had the opportunity to notify the Commissioners of Lunacy of her admission.

Despite a large amount of literature on the subject of asylum life from the staff and lunacy commissioners' point of view, there remain few documented cases of the feelings and views of patients in need of care in these establishments in the nineteenth century. There are accounts from well-educated, private patients about their experiences behind the walls of the asylum, but virtually none from pauper patients. As a result, the story told by Alice Hadfield Petschler following her release from an asylum in 1872 is quite unusual. Alice was one of the first patients to be admitted to Parkside Asylum in Macclesfield, Cheshire in 1871. A subsequent complaint she made against her incarceration provides a unique insight into life behind the walls of this asylum from a patient's point of view.

Case study: Alice Hadfield Petschler

Alice Hadfield Petschler, daughter of John Bennett and his wife Milicent, was born in Glossop, Derbyshire in 1830. In 1854 she married German-born Manchester photographer Helmuth Carl Friedrich Martin Petschler, and the couple, who lived in Gorton, Lancashire had four children – a son Frederic, and three daughters, Millicent, Alice and Elise between 1856 and 1868. Following her husband's early death at the age of 38 in 1869, Mrs Petschler endeavoured to carry on supporting herself and her children with the assistance of her family and friends.

Her sister, Harriet Cuffley, became concerned about her mental wellbeing and in consultation with her brother in law, Dr William Wardlaw Howard, a medical practitioner from Glossop in Derbyshire, arranged for Mrs Petschler to be admitted to Parkside Asylum in Macclesfield. Parkside was a brand new asylum, opened in 1871 and designed to cater predominantly for pauper lunatics, but it also accepted a small number of private patients.

Mrs Petschler was admitted as a pauper patient on 11 November 1871, when it was noted by asylum staff that the death of her husband two years previously had greatly affected her circumstances. Mrs Petschler was diagnosed with 'Delusional Insanity' because she believed her food was being poisoned out of jealousy by people who knew a minister was in love with her and wished to marry her. The case notes reveal that Alice Petschler had followed a minister around for a considerable amount of time and had 'quite persecuted him'. She was given a single room off a female dormitory and was noted to read the Bible a great deal. Alice refused to eat at Parkside claiming she had taken a vow 'not to eat any meal or potatoes as long as she is separated from her children.' She was discharged from Parkside on trial on 20 September 1872.

Mrs Petschler was so horrified by her treatment at Parkside that she wrote about her ordeals and the daily newspapers were only too happy to publish her narrative. The following account was published in the *Birmingham Daily Post* on Monday 23 June 1873.

Mrs Alice Hadfield Petschler, the widow of a well-known Manchester photographer, and whose relatives are people of means and position, was in November 1871, residing at No. 28, The Downs, Bowden, Cheshire about eight miles from Manchester. She carried on the business of her late husband after his death, and maintained herself respectably by the aid of her friends, her business and by letting lodgings, never having applied to the parish for any relief whatever. In October of that year she got into a low nervous state of health, resulting in a slight mental derangement – not, however, sufficiently remarkable to interfere with her photographic business. The symptoms showed that she laboured under a few harmless delusions caused by 'religious mania'. This at least appears to be the case according to a statement of facts appended to the official document signed by the overseer and clergyman upon the strength of which (and the certificate of a medical man that she was a 'person of unsound mind') she was incarcerated. One evening (Saturday November 10, 1871) as she was quietly sitting down to her tea, a cab drove up to the door, some so-called friends announced themselves, and persuaded her, under various pretences, to drive off with them for the ostensible purpose of visiting a doctor, adding that 'she would not be long away'. They took her a long drive, after dark, of fourteen miles towards Macclesfield, where the conveyance drew up at the county asylum. Mrs Petschler writes:-

'When I found I was to be left at the asylum I refused to stop. The doctor summoned three or four nurses, and I was dragged out of the room. I screamed out until they had got me in the corridor and locked the door behind us – I then made a great effort to calm myself for fear I should die – my heart felt as if it would burst. I was taken into a dormitory where there were sixteen lunatics in bed. The horrors of that night I shall never forget – some swearing, some calling dreadful disgusting names, some going into fits, and the night-nurse coming in three or four times. Instead of feeling her a protection she also frightened me – a tall Scotch woman, with a dark lantern. She threw the light on me every time she came in as my bed was near the door. She was very cross with me because I implored her to let me sleep outside the room on the floor, the following morning was Sunday'.

'The patients were frightful-looking objects, dressed in pauper clothes, caps, check aprons, &. I had to wash, and use the same towel and hair-brush after them. Afterwards I had to troop to church with the pauper lunatics and sit with them. There were about fifty-nine patients in the ward I had to sit and take my meals in. Some of them must have been the lowest and most degraded of human beings, and many of them were most repulsive to look at. The nurses treated me as a pauper and used force to me when I refused to submit, telling me I was only a pauper like the rest'.

'On one occasion I refused to take a bath with dirty women round me and two nurses in the room. They fetched the matron, and I told her I was neither helpless nor a lunatic. She told me I must submit to the rules or be forced and ordered them to take me. On another occasion when the boots I had on were worn out, and

had written to tell Mrs. —, who instructed the doctor to get me a pair, the matron wanted me to take off one of my boots, to send to town for a measure. I told her I had some thin slippers in my box, too cold and thin to wear and one of them would surely do instead. As I refused to take off my boot I was thrown on the floor by the nurse and my boot taken off'.

'One fine afternoon I presumed to take a chair out in the airing court, as the two benches were always occupied by the old women. When we were out the door was locked on us for two or three hours. I used to be so tired with walking about, and through not having anywhere to sit down. When it was known that I had taken the chair out, the matron sent a nurse to take the chair from me and bring me in. I refused to go, and seized by two nurses and dragged in. My wrist was painful and swollen for some days after by the rough handling of one of the nurses. They afterwards got two more benches'.

'On another occasion, when I refused to sit at the dinner-table – the dirty cloth, the dirty patients at it, and the smell sickened me – I was seized upon and dragged to it. There was a woman placed in the bedroom I was in who had her leg broken by another patient and had also a sore back. As soon as I had got into bed two nurses used to come to change her sheets and dress her wounds. They lifted her on to the floor. Her groans and screams all night were dreadful to hear and smell left in the room was unbearable. It made me ill. I could not eat, and my not doing so was the only complaint they could make against me'.

'The contents of my dinner plate were often seized upon by the dirty hands of the patients, and my bread was daily handled by them. I was more than once stunned by blows, and knocked down by mad women. One woman took a dislike to me, because the minister spoke to me; she said he was her husband, and three or four times she gave me a blow on my chest and sent me to the floor. Another mad woman gave me such a blow on my face with a shoe that I fell with sickness, my handkerchief was saturated with blood and I was disfigured for two or three weeks'.

'I never required a doctor to attend me the whole of the time I was there. The pain I had suffered from left me a few days after I was in the asylum. I only suffered from heart-ache and sore throat,

caught from sitting near open windows, owing to the smell in the room being unbearable. Many of the patients had not sense enough to attend to themselves. The Christmas holidays came, and my little girl had left school for her first holidays. It had been her first half term (and we had so talked and planned for that time), but I was still kept there. I was nearly broken-hearted. The Midsummer holidays came and Milly from school, and I was still kept there. The doctor had then written to say I might be fetched out. Two months later the doctor went from home with his family for six weeks. The day before he went he wrote again a second time to say I might be taken out. Whilst he was away nearly every day the assistant doctor and the matron on their rounds asked me if I had not yet heard from them, and said it was very strange. The other doctor said the same when he returned'.

'The commissioners came through the ward about four months before I left, and took each patient's name down, I told them – (there were two gentlemen) – I did not consider myself a patient. One of them said, 'But I hear you do not eat your dinner'. I told him I had good reasons for not eating there; I could eat my dinner if I were at home with my children. The first three months, hoping every week I should surely be taken out I did try to eat what was set before me, and worked industriously at all the sewing, marking the house linen and patients' clothes. Once I had some of their dirty linen, stockings and sheets to mark. Towards the last I refused to work and ate very sparingly. The minister asked me to read to the patients and I often did so. I was told by the doctor I could only write to three of my relatives and to my children'.

According to a letter from the medical officer of the asylum, Mrs Petschler was discharged on October 21, 1872, after being a month on trial.

The details of Alice Petschler's treatment caused such a wide sensation that the Committee of Visiting Magistrates of the Asylum immediately conducted an enquiry into the facts of the case. They examined twenty-nine witnesses on oath including two former patients who had been in Parkside at the same time as Mrs Petschler but had since recovered from their mental illness. The other witnesses were asylum employees some of whom had left and moved away from Cheshire. Despite their investigations into her allegations the commissioners were unable to corroborate many of her accusations. They summed up by declaring that 'Mrs Petschler does not appear at any time to have realised the fact that she was insane and required care in an asylum; but she seems to have been mainly and principally aggrieved at having been sent to a *pauper* asylum, and at having to associate with patients beneath herself in station and education.'

The case of Mrs Petschler remained in the press for many years as exaggerated accounts appeared in newspapers. Her sisters, Mrs Cuffley and Mrs Howard, were portrayed in a negative light that resulted in family friction. Alice Petschler died in Withington, Lancashire on 30 October 1897.

While many of Mrs Petschler's complaints were deemed unfounded due to insanity, what was not disputed was the manner in which she was taken to the asylum and the sleeping, washing and meal arrangements that she experienced while she was there. For those admitted to pauper asylums from middle class backgrounds, it was clearly a distressing experience to have to mingle with people they perceived as low class lunatics and imbeciles. But there was no middle class in the asylum system – those who could afford to pay asylum fees were admitted as private patients but those who could not were forced to join the pauper side of the asylum.

Mrs Petschler's description of the sleeping and personal hygiene arrangements at Parkside were not disputed and as this was a new asylum would have been considered relatively luxurious in comparison to older more antiquated buildings. The bedsteads were wooden, constructed of polished birch with straw palliasses and hair mattresses. There were lavatories attached to each dormitory and bathrooms close at hand.

Chapter 11

Asylum Staff

Within the community of each asylum there were communities of patients and of medical, attendant, and establishment staff, who ensured the smooth running of the institution in an efficient, effective and safe manner.

At the head was the medical superintendent who was either a surgeon or physician who lived in the asylum or in a house within the grounds. As well as being the senior medically qualified person at the asylum, he also had responsibility for the administration of the institution and for staff management. Medical superintendents were known as 'alienists'. As the breadth of knowledge and experience of alienists increased during the nineteenth century the field of psychiatry evolved developing into its own specific medical speciality.

Assistant medical officers (AMOs) were junior medical staff who were required to live in the asylum. They were quite often newly qualified, unmarried men undergoing training in treating the insane. On many occasions they made the initial examination and assessment, both physical and mental, of newly admitted patients. They dealt with routine medical problems and emergencies but the medical superintendent oversaw the diagnoses and treatment of mental illnesses. It was the job of the medical superintendent to inform the Lunacy Commissioners of each new admission.

Attendants lived in the asylum and were expected to take part in all the institutional activities and to provide a role model of upright and decent behaviour and moral probity. They had to ensure that they did not use excessive force when dealing with violent or disruptive patients. Any deviation from this could result in disciplinary action, dismissal or even prosecution. An extreme example, where two attendants were held responsible for the manslaughter of a patient, is detailed in Chapter 1. However, there are chronicled cases where asylum staff put their own lives at risk when caring for their patients. On Monday 17 September 1894 two female nurses took a group of fifteen or twenty patients for a walk outside the confines of the asylum – what should have been a pleasant stroll turned out very differently and was reported in the local paper.

When in the dell near the lake, one of them, who was of a suicidal tendency, ran to the lake and jumped in near the bridge, where the water is three or four foot deep. She was immediately followed by one of the nurses, who jumped in after her. A terrible struggle then ensued in the water, and the inmate, getting the mastery, knocked the nurse down in the water, and held her down by standing on her. Seeing this, the other nurse jumped in, and after her a second lunatic, evidently with the desire to assist them. Just at this juncture when their lives were in the most imminent danger, two youths about 16 years of age, came along, and seeing the plight in which they were in, jumped in after them. There were thus six of them in the water at once. The youths eventually managed to get the first lunatic off the nurse, and assisted them all out of the water. Most of them presented a miserable spectacle – especially the inmate who first jumped in, and the nurse after her, who were wet to the skin. Mrs. Frith, of the Cemetery Lodge, kindly assisted all she could in providing dry clothing, and a cab was fetched in which the unfortunate nurse and her unruly patient were conveyed to the Asylum. The nurse lost her keys and one or two other articles, and the lake was afterwards run off, but although a search for them was make by a couple of the male attendants at the Asylum, no trace of them has been found.

Macclesfield Courier, 22 September 1894.

Typically, each asylum had a head male attendant for the male patients and a matron for the female patients, who supervised the day-to-day running of the asylum and reported back to the medical superintendent. The teams of male and female attendants worked long hours and lived with the patients day and night under the same roof. Recruitment adverts for their positions in newspapers indicate how accomplished they needed to be. As well as being able to care for the insane, they were obliged to be literate and were also regularly required to be proficient in a musical

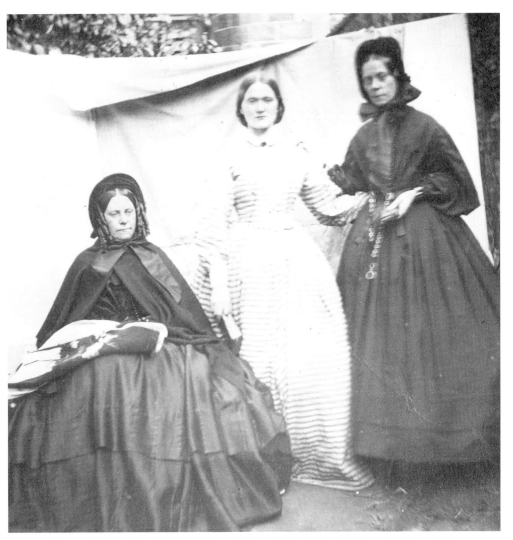

Murray Asylum Perth, 1860. From left to right: Miss Giddings, Matron, Miss Shears, Housekeeper, and Miss Gidding's sister. Courtesy of Dundee University Archive Services.

instrument or a foreign language, and to encourage and participate in the leisure and educational activities of the patients. In the 1890s, Parkside Asylum in Cheshire advertised for an attendant who could play the euphonium and a first violinist at a salary of £30 per annum with uniform, board, lodging and laundry included.

Female attendants were easier to recruit than men because the work was considered to be above that of a domestic servant, which was the highest employment in nineteenth century Britain and Ireland. Many female attendants were recruited from the class of individuals destined for domestic service, which made them ideal for many of the duties required of them in the asylum. Attendants did not merely care for patients, but were also required to keep the asylum clean and tidy and to write comments about the patients in the records. Female attendants rarely stayed in their posts following marriage and there was, therefore, a higher turnover of female staff than male.

Male attendants were more difficult to recruit because of the skills they were required to have. Physical strength was certainly regarded as a positive attribute as was a background in farming or a skilled artisan trade. Male attendants accompanied patients when they worked outdoors and artisan attendants spent half their week in asylum workshops and half their week working in the wards. Former military service personnel found the work conducive due to their regimented former lives, shared accommodation and physical strength. The roles of both male and female attendants were very much a combination of carers, disciplinarians and labourers.

In 1847, the English Commissioners in Lunacy recommended to the Lord Chancellor in their annual report that a Register of Attendants should be maintained in order to verify and keep track of those attendants who worked in lunatic asylums.

Lunatics are placed very much at the mercy of their attendants, it is most desirable to secure, as far as possible, persons of humane and respectable character. In order to promote this object, we have thought it expedient to issue a circular letter, requesting the Superintendent or Proprietor of every Lunatic Establishment to forward to us the names of all male and female attendants employed by him, and to transmit notice upon all future occasions whenever any attendant shall be engaged or dismissed, or shall quit the asylum, together with the cause of every dismissal; to the intent that a Central Register may be established at our Office.

Report of the Commissioners in Lunacy,
to the Lord Chancellor. 1847

The Register was considered an important aspect of maintaining a high standard of care within asylums, and male and female attendants were also encouraged to take nursing examinations to prove their competency. In 1884, the first edition of *The Handbook for the Instruction of Attendants on the Insane* was published to provide guidelines for institutions and attendants. It was an early attempt to educate attendants about diseases of the mind and their management. It also provided rules for their guidance of everyday experience in an asylum to enable them to do their work with greater intelligence and watchfulness. The book contained chapters on nursing the sick and caring for the insane, as well as guidance on general behaviour. A training scheme for attendants began in 1891 and those who completed the course, after a minimum of two years' experience of working in an asylum, were provided with a Certificate of Proficiency in Nursing the Insane and allowed to use the post nominal MPA (Medico-Psychological Association). The qualification was highly esteemed by the attendants but did not provide them with additional pay or other working benefits.

The asylum also had an establishment of additional staff who specialised in certain trades. They worked in, and helped run, the laundry, kitchens, gardens and farms of the asylum. Others were responsible for the running and maintenance of the buildings and equipment. Many of these skilled tradesmen provided workshops for the patients and this allowed many of the male patients to continue working in the occupations they had prior to admission to the asylum. Similarly, female patients, many of whom had been domestic servants, housewives or seamstresses, were encouraged to continue with domestic-type duties.

Chaplains were present in asylums but remained somewhat in a position of isolation, away from the day-to-day running of the asylum, and with no close ties to others in the same profession due to the distance between them. An 'Asylum Chaplain's Column' began to be published in the *British Journal of Psychiatry* from 1893 as a way of providing a community spirit to others who held the same position.

Chaplains were inevitably part of the Established Church, a situation which caused difficulties for many patients of the Roman Catholic faith. In the 1870s, while consultations were taking place for a fourth asylum for the county of Lancaster, it was proposed that the new building should be used to house the county's Roman Catholic lunatic population of whom it was estimated there were over 820 individuals. This plan was supported by the Home Secretary who voiced his concern over the lack of instruction available to those of non-established faiths. Despite this however, the asylum remained open to all creeds and a Catholic priest visited the asylum whenever he was needed.

Chaplains regularly visited the wards – in particular the infirmary – and were free to hold prayers as they wished. The majority of asylums had dedicated churches – although many of these were built after the asylum as an addition to the provision for patients. Patients were encouraged to participate in church services but remained segregated from each other. An asylum report from Glasgow Royal Asylum dated 1821 stated:

> *The chapel must be large enough to accommodate about 100 auditors. The means of separating the males from the females, so that they shall not be able to see each other, while they may have it in their power to see the clergyman; and also the means of separating the patients of higher ranks from their inferiors.*

In 1857 the Commissioners Report on James Murray Asylum, Perth declared that:

> *The two sexes sit apart, but in view of each other ... a partition completely divides the room into two compartments, leaving half of the pulpit in each.*

Whilst the chaplain was head of a spiritual community, that community did not resemble an ordinary parish. Many asylum chaplains were young and unmarried and their work in an asylum was quite often the first post they held following ordination.

An example of the list of staff employed at Glasgow Royal Asylum in 1855 is given in the table on the next page, with their rates of pay and allowances. Female staff were paid much less than their male counterparts.

Medical and other Officers, Attendants and Establishment.
Glasgow Royal Asylum. 1855.
Number of patients: 87 private; 329 paupers; total 416.

Official	Annual Salary	Allowances
Physician superintendent	£500	A house in the Institution, with coals, gas, water and washing, garden vegetables except potatoes.
Medical Assistants x 2	£80 each	Board, washing and lodging in the Institution.
Superintendent of ladies	£100	Board, washing and lodging in the Institution.
Steward	£110	A house, with coals, gas, water and washing, garden vegetables except potatoes.
Master of works	£100	ditto
Gardener and farm overseer	£70	ditto
Surgeon paid according to number of visits, operations, &c. Average for last 3 years	£28	
Treasurer and secretary	£300	
Chaplain	£60	

Attendants	Wages p.a.	Allowances
MALES Principal attendant	£42	All the attendants have, beside their wages, board, washing, and lodging in the Institution
Attendant x 1	£34	
Attendants x 2	£32 ea.	
Attendants x 11	£30 ea.	
Attendants x 8	£26 ea.	
FEMALES Principal Attendant	£40	
Attendants x 2	£17 each	
Attendants x 11	£15 each	
Attendants x 3	£12 each	

Establishment	Wages p.a.	Allowances
MALES Coachman	£46 12s. 0d.	A house, with coals, gas, water and washing, garden vegetables except potatoes.
Gate-keeper	£54 12s. 0d.	ditto
Store-keeper	£40	Board, washing and lodging in the Institution.
Baker	£49 8s. 0d.	ditto
Assistant baker	£19 10s. 0d.	ditto

Gardener	£40	ditto
Stoker	£33	ditto
Coal porter	£15	ditto
Door-keeper	£30	ditto
Farm servants x 3	£28 each	ditto
Farm servant x 1	£19	ditto
Tailor	£26	ditto
Shoemaker	£30	ditto
Joiners x 3	£62 8s. each	These tradesmen act as attendants every alternate Sunday, for which they are allowed 6s each and food.
Plumber	£62 8s.	ditto
Blacksmith	£62 8s.	ditto
Mason	£70 4s.	ditto
Engineer	£52	No extra allowance
Labourer	£39	The labourer relieves the engineer every alternate Sunday, for which he is allowed 2s. 6d. and food.
FEMALES Principal laundress	£18	Board, washing and lodging in the Institution.
Laundresses x 2	£14 each	ditto
Laundresses x 4	£12 each	ditto
Dressmaker	£15	ditto
Upholsteress	£15 10s.	ditto
Portress and housemaid	£14	ditto

Portress and housemaid	£12	ditto
Housemaid	£12	ditto
Housemaid	£9	ditto
Cook	£16	ditto
Cooks x 2	£12 each	ditto

As most of the asylum staff lived in, the decennial censuses give further information about them including their name, age, gender, marital status and place of birth. An example of this is the 1891 census for the West Riding District Lunatic Asylum at Wakefield. This was a large asylum and on census night – 5 April 1891 – there were 645 male patients and 673 females.

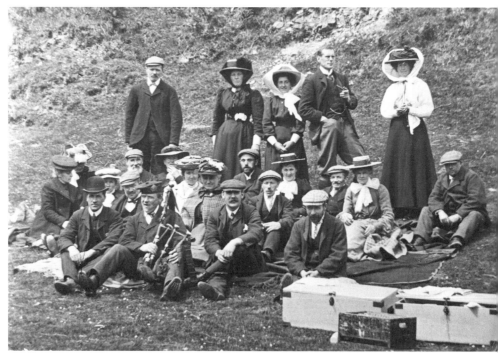

Staff outing. Montrose Royal Asylum. Courtesy of Dundee University Archive Services.

ASYLUM STAFF

The medical superintendent, Dr William Bevan Lewis from Cardigan, Wales lived in a separate residence in the asylum grounds with his wife and mother and had his own cook and housemaid. Within the asylum, he was supported by three assistant medical officers – two physicians and a surgeon. The nursing team comprised a chief female officer, a head nurse and sixty-five other nurses. Of these, one was married, another was a widow, and the remainder were single women, mostly in their twenties or early thirties, with the majority being born in Yorkshire or Lancashire. The chief attendant was a 73-year-old widower who had his daughter and a grandson living with him and the deputy chief male attendant was married with a young son staying in the asylum. There were a further nineteen male attendants, all single. The farm bailiff lived with his wife and six children on the asylum farm. Other asylum staff listed include a storekeeper, a butler, a lodge keeper, an engineer, a painter and decorator, three cooks, a dairy maid, and two kitchen maids. There were also four passage maids. The asylum had a live-in laundress with a team of seven laundry maids.

Chapter 12

The Criminal Lunatic

One seminal incident in 1800 – a threat to the life of King George III – changed the way in which criminals who were considered to be insane at the time of committing their offence(s) were subsequently dealt with by the judicial systems within the United Kingdom. The perpetrator of the attempted murder of King George, James Hadfield, who was also charged with treason, was acquitted by reason of 'insanity'.

England and Wales
James Hadfield (1771–1841) had been a cavalry officer of exemplary conduct and respect who had served in the British Army in Flanders in the 15th King's Regiment of Light Hussars. In 1794 he received multiple head injuries during operations at Tourcoing in France. Several blows from a sabre to the side of his head, followed by a cut to his left cheek, forced Hadfield off his horse and into a ditch on the battlefield. Hadfield was presumed dead but subsequently found by two French officers after the battle who took him to a house full of dead bodies. The following day, after being provided with milk and water, Hadfield walked to a British wagon from where he was transferred to a military hospital to receive treatment for his head wounds. Hadfield's experiences in battle and the trauma to his head and face left his mind in a very deranged state and he began to suffer delusions of persecution and threatened to kill his own child. Hadfield was honourably discharged from the army in 1796 due to insanity; he never fully recovered from the trauma of his war experiences and became deluded, believing that in order to save the world, he must die at the hands of the British Government. In order to guarantee this fate he decided to assassinate the king.

On the evening of 15 May 1800, Hadfield fired a pistol at George III as he entered the Royal Box at the Drury Lane Theatre in London during the playing of the National Anthem. Hadfield's aim was poor and he missed his target by over 12ins. This event, and the resulting court case, highlighted the inadequacies of the law at that time and provided a major catalyst in establishing the 1800 *Criminal Lunatics Act* and the 1800 *Treason Act* which were both proposed by the prosecution four days after Hadfield's trial.

Prior to 1800, individuals who were acquitted of crimes by reason of insanity were set free and released in to the safe-keeping of their families because there was no law under which they could be detained. This situation was radically altered after Hadfield's trial and the *Criminal Lunatics Act* ensured that those guilty of treason, murder, or felony, who were deemed to be insane, should be sent to a suitable asylum facility. The terms of the 1800 Act stated that:

> *If the jury shall find that such person was insane at the time of the committing such offence, the court before whom such trial shall be had, shall order such person to be kept in strict custody, in such place and in such manner as to the court shall seem fit, until His Majesty's pleasure shall be known.*

This Act received Royal Assent on 28 July 1800.

Many insane prisoners were sent to the Bethlehem Hospital in London and state funding was obtained to build additional accommodation for this new category of patient. At this stage it was not considered important to build a specific asylum for criminal lunatics and they were, in effect, allowed to enter an establishment where vulnerable insane patients were also housed. It would take another assassination attempt and a murder before the legislation was further amended.

In 1843, Daniel McNaughton (1813–65), a lathe-worker from Glasgow, travelled to London determined to kill the British prime minister, Sir Robert Peel (1788–1850), as he was possessed by paranoid delusions that government spies were following him. Fortunately for Sir Robert, McNaughton mistook Peel's private secretary, Edward Drummond (1792–1843), for Peel and it was Drummond who was shot in the back and subsequently died five days later. After a lengthy trial at Middlesex Central Criminal Court, McNaughton was acquitted, absolved of liability because he was considered to be insane and, as a result, could not be considered accountable for his actions. This verdict outraged the public, and ensured that insanity was further defined in cases of criminal law. Following a House of Lords review it was determined that the law had to prove whether the defendant knew what he was doing at the time of the crime and, if so, that he was aware that it was wrong. Following this ruling, criminals deemed to be insane were treated differently within the judicial system. McNaughton spent the rest of his life in an asylum, predominantly Bethlehem, but died in Broadmoor in 1865 of heart and kidney disease.

Lord Shaftesbury motioned the House of Commons in 1852 to build a separate facility for the detention of criminal lunatics in England and Wales. He produced reams of testimony from medical superintendents of several asylums in order to make the case that allowing criminals to be housed with vulnerable insane patients was not beneficial. He was also aware, and very much approved, of the new facility at Dundrum outside Dublin in Ireland which had opened in 1850 for the reception of the criminally insane. His list of the principal reasons assigned by the superintendents of asylums, for the non-association of criminal lunatics with ordinary lunatic patients is provided below.

It is unjust to ordinary patients to associate them with persons branded with crime. The lunatic is generally very sensitive, and both he and his friends feel aggrieved and degraded by the association. The moral effect is bad. The conduct of criminal patients is frequently very violent; their habits and language, the result of previous habits, are frequently offensive, and their influence on other patients injurious and pernicious. By the fact of stricter custody being required, and greater responsibility felt for criminal patients, the general classification of patients in an asylum is interrupted, and the improved discipline and proper treatment of other patients interfered with; the expense is also increased for safe keeping. The common delusion that an asylum is a prison is strengthened by lunatic patients being compelled to associate with persons who have been in prison; and, in fact, higher walls than those ordinarily in use have been considered necessary (and in one case erected) for the security of criminal lunatics associated with other patients. The association is injurious even to the criminal patients. It exposes them to taunts from the other patients, and the stricter confinement imposed on themselves irritates them. They are irritated also when other patients are liberated, and they left in confinement. When criminal patients are confided in (in the same way as other patients), it is generally found that they are unworthy of trust; that they try to escape and induce others to do so, and that insubordination and dissatisfaction are generally produced by their influence. The criminal patients concentrate attention on themselves, and attract an undue share of care and supervision from the attendants. Cases of simulated insanity are (supposed to be) not infrequent with patients received as criminal lunatics. In those cases the patients are mostly patients of the worst character. They create discontent among the other patients, and oppress those who are weaker than themselves, and they generally try to escape. Patients of the criminal class, even when unsound at the time of committing the offence, possess criminal propensities, and in some cases their insanity has been caused by vicious habits. The most efficient remedy for this state of things, would, in my opinion, be the establishment of a State asylum for the separate care and custody of those who were termed criminal lunatics; and for this I have the approbation of almost all the medical superintendents and persons most conversant with lunacy throughout the United Kingdom.

A specialist facility was clearly required and, as a result, the concept of Broadmoor was born. The *Criminal Lunatic Asylums Act* of 1860 allowed the government to build a specialist facility so that the classification of patients should not be confused and those deemed to be dangerous should be kept away from those considered likely of a cure. As a result Broadmoor was founded.

Broadmoor Hospital for the Criminally Insane was built in the village of Crowthorne, Berkshire in 1863. Designed by Sir Joshua Jebb (1793–1863), a military engineer who had previously designed two prisons, it was constructed using labour provided by convicts from Parkhurst Prison on the Isle of Wight. In keeping with asylum legislation, it was situated in attractive countryside in a large, clean and spacious building close to a railway station for the ease of transferring patients.

The first patients to be transferred from Bethlehem in London in 1863 were eight women. Of these, six had killed or wounded their children using a variety of different methods. Numbers of admissions fluctuated

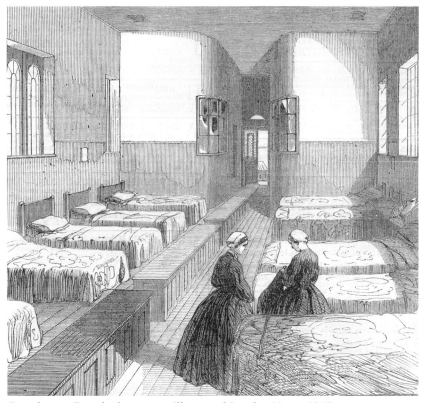

Broadmoor. Female dormitory. Illustrated London News, 1867.

Broadmoor. Day room for Male Patients. Illustrated London News, 1867.

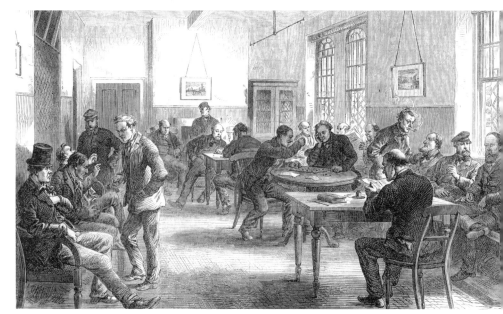

slightly but there were generally about 500 patients in the asylum at any one time. They were sent from all over England and Wales and were from a combination of all social classes. Many never received visitors due to the huge distances involved in travelling to Berkshire.

Case study: William Thicknesse-Tuchet

One of the earliest patients was the Honourable William Ross Thicknesse-Tuchet, third and youngest son of George, the twentieth Lord Audley (1783–1837). Tuchet deliberately shot a gunsmith, Thomas Smith of High Holborn, in the back – an action he claimed to have done on purpose because he wished to be hanged. Twenty-two year old Tuchet was tried at London's Central Criminal Court, The Old Bailey, on 21 October 1844 and found to be not guilty due to unsound mind. He was initially detained at Her Majesty's Pleasure at Bethlem Asylum, London and was later transferred to Broadmoor on 23 March 1864. He died there classified as a pauper patient on 1 December 1893.

Case study: Margaret Hibbert

On 5 June 1885, Margaret Hibbert of Moss Side, Manchester, drowned her two young sons, James aged 5 and John aged 3, in the family bath and then laid them out in bed covered by a sheet. She was tried for murder at Manchester Summer Assizes, but was deemed to be unfit to plead due to insanity.

Margaret had already spent time in an asylum because of her repeated verbal desire to end not only the lives of her children, but also her own. Margaret had been admitted to Parkside Asylum in Macclesfield, Cheshire in July 1884 only ten weeks after the birth of her youngest son. Expressing a wish to kill herself and her two children Margaret was diagnosed with 'lactational insanity' – one diagnosis in the spectrum of post-puerperal insanity – and she was admitted to the asylum. Margaret was prescribed chloral hydrate and potassium bromide to help her sleep because she suffered delusions, ate very little, and expressed a desire to die because she was wicked. Her behaviour was aggressive, and when she attempted to strangle another patient she was placed in a padded room for her own safety and the safety of others.

In June 1885, Margaret Hibbert's husband removed her from the asylum against the advice of the asylum medical superintendent who did not believe she had recovered. His thoughts were well founded as two days later she murdered both her children and attempted to strangle herself. The asylum medical superintendent, Thomas Steele Sheldon, gave evidence in court expressing his concern that he had feared there would be a relapse of Margaret's fragile mental health and did not believe that she had been ready to be 'relieved' from asylum care. However, Margaret's husband had signed a declaration stating that he would be responsible for her actions and so she was free to return home.

At her trial there was no doubt in the minds of the judge or jury that Margaret was not responsible for her actions and instead of receiving the death penalty for her crime, she was sentenced to be confined in strict custody at Her Majesty's pleasure. She was detained in Broadmoor.

Case study: Joseph Waller

Another Broadmoor inmate was Joseph Waller, a 24-year-old labourer convicted of the double murder of Edward and Elizabeth Ellis in Chislehurst, Kent on 31 October 1880. The murder was a particularly brutal attack on two elderly people whom Ellis had previously worked for.

Joseph Waller left The Five Bells public house in St Mary Cray, Kent, with a loaded revolver in his pocket and claimed to be tempted by 'an uncontrollable impulse to commit a desperate deed.' He went to the home of Edward Ellis, his former employer and a gamekeeper, and, firing a shot, shouted that there were poachers about. Mr Ellis came out of the cottage with a truncheon and a lantern and accompanied Waller into the woods, where he was shot in the head and clubbed with his own truncheon. Waller returned to the cottage to tell Mrs Ellis that her husband wanted her and as he led her towards her husband's body, he shot and bludgeoned her to death too.

Waller's Irish mother, Catherine, testified in court that she could prove her son was not sane. Waller had been a police constable with the Metropolitan force previously stationed at Worship Street – Catherine claimed she had been scared of him all her life and knew that he should have been in an asylum. An accident during his time with the police service had worsened his condition and she felt that he should have been in St Luke's Asylum. An examination from the medical superintendent at Colney Hatch Asylum in Middlesex confirmed that Waller was not sane and he was sent to Broadmoor in 1881. He remained there until his death on 10 April 1923.

Case study: John Biggs

John Biggs was an 18-year-old millwright who had cut the throat of his sweetheart, Mary Ann Bromwich, with a razor in Evington, Leicester on 19 June 1879. Biggs confessed to killing her and admitted that he had contemplated suicide as a result of his crime. Biggs suffered from epilepsy and mania, both his parents and a maternal uncle were also in an asylum and his brother was considered to be an imbecile.

During cross-examination at his trial, Biggs stated that Mary Ann had not suffered any pain from her fatal injury. He was found guilty and sentenced to death. The date of the execution was set for 5 August 1879 but the defence pleaded for mercy, claiming Biggs was suffering from 'heredity insanity and a fit of acute mania' having been parted from his sweetheart after enlistment. The death sentence was commuted on the grounds of insanity and Biggs was sent to Broadmoor. He remained there until his death.

Not all the patients at Broadmoor were adults. Children were also admitted if their crimes were considered serious and they had a mental health disorder.

Case study: Robert Coombes

In 1895, 13-year-old Robert Allen Coombes a plater's helper of Cave Road, Plaistow, London and his 11-year-old brother, Nathaniel George Coombes, were charged at West Ham Police Court with the murder of their mother Emily. The post-mortem showed that she had been stabbed in the left breast by a dagger knife. The boys concealed her death and carried on as if nothing had happened, very much ignoring the gravity of the situation they were in. They went to Lord's Cricket Ground and informed the neighbours that their mother had gone to Liverpool to visit her family. Emily's body lay undiscovered in her bedroom for ten days. The boys were charged with her murder but Nathaniel was discharged because Robert admitted purchasing the knife and committing the stabbing.

The trial of Robert Coombes took place at the Old Bailey in London. Robert's father, also called Robert Coombes, who was away at sea when the murder took place, was questioned about insanity within the family. He stated that there was none in his family but his wife had been an excitable woman and his son Robert had marks on the side of his head from a forceps delivery and regularly complained of severe headaches.

George Edward Walker, the medical officer for Holloway and Newgate prisons, stated on evidence that Robert was:

> *singing and whistling, and was very impertinent to the officers – he has complained of pains in the head on two or three occasions – he told me he had suffered from them more or less all his life – there is a distinct scar on his right temple, and on very careful examination I noticed also a very faint scar just in front of his left ear – those scars might have been caused by instruments used at the time of his birth – the brain is always compressed more or less when instruments are used, which will occasionally affect the brain.*

George Walker was of the opinion that Robert Coombes was suffering from cerebral excitement:

> *It was peculiar, he appeared in very great glee at being about to be brought here to be tried, his manner was peculiar, but you would hardly say he was suffering from very great excitement that day, he thought it would be a splendid sight, and he was looking forward to it, he said he would wear his best clothes and have his boots well polished, then he began to talk about his cats, from having been very talkative he suddenly became very silent and burst into tears. I asked him why he was crying, and he said because he wanted his cats and his mandolin. I have his letter, which was handed to me on Sunday, which appears to be written by an insane person.*

Letter addressed to Mr. Shaw, 583, Barking Road, Plaistow, Essex, from R. A. Coombes, HM Prison, Holloway, 14 September 1895:

> *Dear Mr. Shaw, I received your letter on last Tuesday. I think I will get hung, but I do not care as long as I get a good breakfast before they hang me. If they do not hang me I think I will commit suicide. That will do just as well. I will strangle myself. I hope you are all well. I go up on Monday to the Old Bailey to be tried. I hope you will be there I think they will sentence me to die. If they do I will call all the witnesses liars.*
>
> *I remain, yours affectionately, R. A. Coombes.*

The bottom of the letter contained a series of images – 'Scene I', going to the Scaffold, a drawing of a gibbet and two figures being pushed forward by another; over the last figure was written, 'Executioner'. 'Scene II', a drawing of a gibbet with a person being hanged, and the words, 'Goodbye' issuing from his mouth, and the writing, 'Here goes nothing!'

Robert also wrote a will, which was shown to the assembled court. It read:

> *My will:*
> *To Dr. Walker, £3,000; to Mr. Payne, £2,000; to Mr. Shaw, £5,000;*
> *to my father, £60,000; to all the warders, £300 a piece. Signed, R.*
> *Coombes, Chairman, Solicitor.*
> *P.S. Excuse the crooked scaffold, I was too heavy, I bent it; I leave*
> *you £5,000'.*

The letter strengthened the opinion of Robert's mental condition and indicated insanity. He was diagnosed with homicidal mania.

Robert Coombes was initially sent to Holloway Prison where the medical officer noted periodic attacks of mania. He was moved by train to Broadmoor accompanied by two warders; the press stated that he returned the glances of his fellow passengers with a careless smile as he made the journey.

Coombes thrived in Broadmoor where he was one of the youngest patients. He joined the brass band and played cricket in the first XI. Coombes was lucky enough to be discharged from Broadmoor in 1912 and emigrated to Australia where, in Sydney in September 1914, he enlisted in the 45th Battalion of the Australian Imperial Force. He served at Gallipoli and on 12 October 1916 he was made Band Sergeant. His name was mentioned in British and Australian newspapers when he was awarded the Military Medal on 27 October 1916. His brother Nathaniel also emigrated to Australia and served in the Navy during both World Wars. Robert Coombes died in New South Wales on 7 May 1949.

In England and Wales, not all criminal lunatics were admitted to Broadmoor. In many ways this institution was reserved for the most difficult and challenging patients. Many individuals guilty of less serious crimes and with shorter sentences were maintained either in a local prison or transferred to a local asylum. Criminal lunatics such as prostitute Mary Monaghan were transferred from gaols to asylums if their behaviour was considered dangerous.

Case studies: Mary Monaghan and Mary Ann Wilson
Mary Monaghan, a 21-year-old epileptic prostitute, was sentenced to three months hard labour for drunkenness and wilful damage in 1883. Many epileptics were considered to be 'dangerous' when they were having seizures as their behaviour changed and they often displayed aggressive tendencies. Mary was held at Knutsford Gaol and her seizures increased. As a result she spent the rest of her sentence in Macclesfield Asylum in Cheshire. On admission to the asylum she was described as 'not actively insane'. She proved to be quiet and industrious, and continued to show no signs of insanity. On 21 September 1883, a certificate signed by two medical officers declaring her to be sane was sent to the Home Secretary. On 9 October 1883, she was given an unconditional discharge and released from the asylum vowing to lead a more sober lifestyle.

Mary Ann Wilson was 23 years old when she was admitted to Parkside Asylum from prison in January 1881 suffering from epilepsy and mania. The case notes describe her as 'having the physiognomy suggestive of congenital weakness and is probably a moral imbecile.' Mary Ann claimed to be a domestic servant but the prison records state that she was 'a prostitute, a rogue and a vagabond.' She had to be carefully watched while in the asylum as she always tried to escape and her behaviour was violent and dangerous. Mary was eventually discharged into the community in May 1881, having been in the asylum for four months. There is no suggestion that she was re-admitted.

Scotland
In Scotland criminal lunatics were housed in the General Prison in Perth from the mid-nineteenth century. The bleak and gloomy building chosen for them had originally been used to detain French prisoners-of-war during the Napoleonic campaigns in France and Iberia at the beginning of that century. It was converted in 1846 into a 'Criminal Lunatics Unit' on two floors and took its first inmates in October 1846.

As in England, the main instigators of the changes to the system were medical superintendents who objected to 'the insane being associated with persons who had been charged with committing violent and heinous crimes.' It was believed that a prison asylum that could ensure the close and safe custody of the most dangerous class of lunatics was needed.

Case study: John Laurie – the Arran Murderer of 1889

John Watson Laurie (1864–1930), a pattern-maker from Glasgow, was one of the longest serving prisoners in Scotland – a sentence he served at Greenock, Peterhead and Perth Prisons from 1893 onwards, before finally being admitted to the Criminal Lunacy Department at Perth. In July 1889 Laurie befriended a young London clerk called Edwin Rose (1857–89) travelling on the steamer from Rothesay to the Isle of Arran for a holiday. Laurie invited Rose to share his accommodation on the island. Whilst hillwalking up Goatfell, Arran's highest peak, Laurie allegedly murdered Rose then buried his body under some rocks. It was nearly two weeks before the body of Rose was discovered, by which time Laurie had fled to Liverpool. Laurie was not apprehended until 3 September 1893. He was tried and convicted of murder at the High Court of Judiciary at Edinburgh on 9 November 1893. Despite claiming innocence, Laurie was sentenced to death. The Lord Chief Justice pronounced that Laurie would:

> be carried from the bar to the Prison of Edinburgh thence to be forthwith transmitted to the Prison of Greenock therein to be detained till the thirtieth day of November current, and upon that day between the hours of eight and ten o'clock in the forenoon, within the walls of the said prison by the hands of the common executioner, to be hanged by the neck upon a gibbet until he be dead, and his body thereafter to be buried within the walls of the said prison of Greenock.

Laurie had attempted suicide by cutting his throat with a razor immediately prior to his arrest. On 29 November 1889, the day before his planned execution, Laurie was awarded a conditional pardon by Queen Victoria and the sentence was commuted to one of penal servitude for life. He was transferred initially to Perth Penitentiary to undergo nine month's solitary confinement before being sent to Peterhead Prison where he was forced to work hard labour breaking stones in a quarry. In 1893 Laurie made an attempt to escape from a working party but was quickly recaptured, flogged with thirty strokes of the birch rod, and placed in leg-irons for six months. From 1902 onwards the Medical Officers at Peterhead Prison reported to the Commissioners of Prisons that Laurie was insane with paranoid delusions and enfeeblement of mind. However, it was not until 1910 that Laurie was moved to the Criminal Lunatic Department at Perth Prison. He died there in 1930.

Ireland

The 1821 *Lunacy (Ireland) Act* provided that criminal lunatics – being persons 'acquitted on the ground of insanity of treason, murder, or other offences; to persons indicted and found insane at the time of their arraignment, or brought before any criminal court to be discharged for want of prosecution, appearing insane' would be detained in asylums at the pleasure of His Majesty or the Lord Lieutenant.

The 1838 *Criminal Lunatics (Ireland) Act* applied to persons 'apprehended under circumstances denoting a derangement of mind, and a purpose of committing an indictable crime; to persons who have become insane under sentence of imprisonment or transportation; or under any warrant in default of surety to keep the peace'. This Act became commonly known as the 'Dangerous Lunatics Act' and was much abused. Such patients would initially be committed to a gaol and later transferred to an asylum.

Dr Francis White (1787–1859), as Inspector of Prisons, gave evidence to the House of Lords Select Committee on the State of the Lunatic Poor in Ireland in 1843, in support of a central criminal lunatic institution:

Solid objections exist to criminal lunatics being received into District Asylums which were never intended for prisons. As there is a want of room for pauper lunatics, it would save expense to remove all the criminal lunatics to one spot.

Francis White became one of the first two Inspectors of Lunacy in Ireland in January 1846.

Subsequently, the 1845 *Central Criminal Lunatic Asylum (Ireland) Act* directed that there should only be one central asylum for insane persons charged with offences in Ireland. As a result Dundrum Asylum for the Criminal Insane was established. It was the Irish equivalent of Broadmoor and pre-dated it by thirteen years. The decision to build the facility was made after the murder of Edward Drummond, the Private Secretary to Prime Minister Sir Robert Peel in 1843. Peel had previously been Chief Secretary for Ireland from 1812 until 1818. As mentioned earlier, a special asylum with its own infirmary was opened in Dundrum village on the outskirts of Dublin in 1850. It had room for eighty men and forty women. As would later occur at Broadmoor, the most dangerous and difficult of patients were transferred to Dundrum first with a priority given to anyone who had committed murder. The treatment of patients was of the moral kind and as with other asylums, Dundrum was surrounded by acres of land. Patients worked at their trades, read books and were provided with various activities. The use of restraint and seclusion was restricted to the most violent patients. Lord Shaftesbury viewed the asylum as a positive step forwards, proving that the disassociation of criminal and ordinary lunatics was beneficial.

The 1883 *Trial of Lunatics (Ireland) Act* allowed for the verdict for a convicted person proven guilty but found to be insane at the time of any crime, including murder, to be 'guilty but insane'.

Case study: William Stewart

Captain William Stewart was a mass murderer who killed seven of his crew on a ship returning from Barbados that arrived in Cork Harbour in 1828.

When the transport schooner *Mary Russell* docked at Cobh Harbour, Cork, on 25 June 1828, the harbour-master discovered the bodies of seven murdered crewmembers on board and two other seriously injured seamen. One of the dead was his own brother, James Gould Raynes. The captain of the *Mary Russell*, William Stewart, an experienced navigator and a well-respected, pious man considered to be a pillar of local society, had become psychotic on the voyage back to Ireland from Barbados and was suffering paranoid delusions that the crew were planning a mutiny and intended to kill him. His insane answer was to call them one by one into his saloon, tie them up and subsequently beat their brains out with a crowbar or an axe, or kill them by shooting them in the head with a harpoon.

At a coroner's inquest in Cork the following day Dr Thomas Sharpe testified:

There were seven human beings with their sculls so battered that scarcely a vestige of them was left for recognition, with a frightful mess of coagulated blood – all strewed about the cabin, and nearly a hundredweight of cords binding their bodies to strong iron bolts. ... Some of the bodies were bound round about six places, and with several coils of rope round their necks.

The coroner's court jury's verdict on William Stewart was that 'several sailors and passengers were killed by the hands of Captain William Stewart being insane and for some days before in a state of mental derangement.'

William Stewart was tried by an Admiralty Court convened at Cork Assizes on 11 August 1828 for the capital charge of the murder of James Raynes on the high seas about 100 leagues off the coast of Ireland. The jury's verdict, directed by the judge, was 'not guilty having committed the act while labouring under mental derangement.' Stewart's sentence was 'that he be kept in close confinement during life, or during his Majesty's pleasure.' Stewart was committed initially to the City Gaol of Cork, and thereafter to Cork Lunatic Asylum. He was transferred to the Dundrum Asylum for the Criminal Insane shortly after it opened in 1850, where he died in 1873.

Case study: Catherine Wynn
In Sligo in 1893, another remarkable event occurred. Catherine Wynn, a 35-year-old Catholic married woman, drowned her three children in a bath of boiling water. Catherine then tried to kill herself by putting her head into the same bath of boiling water. She was deemed not responsible for her actions due to insanity and was sent to the Central Criminal Asylum at Dundrum in County Dublin as a 'criminal lunatic'. Catherine did not recover mentally and died in Dundrum.

There are similarities in this case study to the English one previously described – that of Margaret Hibbert in Manchester.

Actions and events that occurred in the nineteenth century helped shape not only asylums, but also the future of those deemed to be criminally insane. Following the assassination of Edward Drummond by Daniel McNaughton and the subsequent change to the law, 'The McNaughton Rules' were created to protect those considered to be of unsound mind. They remain in force to this day.

Chapter 13

Imbeciles and Idiots

"OUT!, thou silly moon-struck elf;
Back, poor fool, and hide thyself!"
This is what the wise ones say,
Should the idiot cross their way,
But if we would closely mark,
We should see him not all dark;
We should find we must not scorn
The teaching of the idiot-born.

Eliza Cook (1818–89), English Poet and Author.

From as early as the thirteenth century there was a clearly defined legal difference established through the judiciary of England between idiots and lunatics. This distinction was made because of the Crown's rights over land inheritance and the statute *De Praerogativa Regis* (of the Royal Prerogative) dating from the time of Edward I (1239–1307), who became King of England, Lord of Ireland and Duke of Aquitaine in 1272. This statute protected the estates of those people who, by a natural progress of mental decay, 'lost their minds'.

Idiots, who in the early days were termed 'natural fools', were seen as having a congenital and permanent condition involving an absence of understanding. Lunatics, on the other hand, also termed persons *non compos mentis*, acquired their lack of reasoning after birth and could have lucid intervals when their mental thought process appeared to be rational. The altered state of mind of lunatics was considered in legal terms to be a temporary illness. The Crown held Royal Prerogative over the guardianship or 'wardship' of the lands of natural fools, taking all the revenues from their estates but at the same time providing for their sustenance. The lands were returned to the idiot's heirs on his death. For those individuals who were declared *non compos mentis,* however, the reigning monarch protected the lunatic's estate and maintained him and his family with estate revenues throughout his illness. All profits from estate revenues reverted to the lunatic or his heirs on his recovery or his death.

By the fifteenth century 'idiot', rather than 'natural fool', had become the preferred term. Thereafter the new category of 'imbecile' was developed in addition to the terms 'idiot' and 'lunatic'. Imbeciles were people who had acquired a permanent cognitive impairment after birth – maybe from causes such as a traumatic brain injury, encephalitis, meningitis, or poisoning by toxins. Their disabilities, although permanent, were generally not considered quite as profound as those of idiots.

The 1845 *Lunatics Act* defined mental incapacity in three ways.

- 'Lunatics', who were temporarily incapacitated but had lucid intervals;
- 'idiots', who had a congenital incapacity with no intervals of sanity; and
- 'persons of unsound mind', who had acquired their incapacity as a result of injury or illness.

Up until the mid-nineteenth century, imbeciles and idiots would have been cared for first by their family, or failing that, by neighbours or through their local community. The terms 'idiots' and 'imbeciles' remained prevalent into the twentieth century. Today they would be recognised as people with learning disabilities and the previous contemporary terminology is now considered to be derogatory, insulting and offensive. The first residential and educational institution for idiots in England was founded at Bath, Somerset, in 1846 by Miss Charlotte White (b. 1820), daughter of Major General Martin White of the Bengal Army. When her establishment opened in April 1846 as the *Bath Institute for Idiot Children and those of Weak Intellect,* it had a resident matron, two rooms and just three pupils. The pupils had all been ill-treated and neglected by their families. In 1851, the Institute, now with eighteen pupils, moved to larger premises. It was a small operation with good intentions. The Bath Institute only had up to thirty students at a time, but went on to care for about 200 children before merging with the Magdalen Charity in 1887 to become part of the Magdalen Hospital School at Rockhall House, Bath.

Another charitable institution in England, *The National Asylum for Idiots*, was established at Park House, Highgate, London, in 1847. This

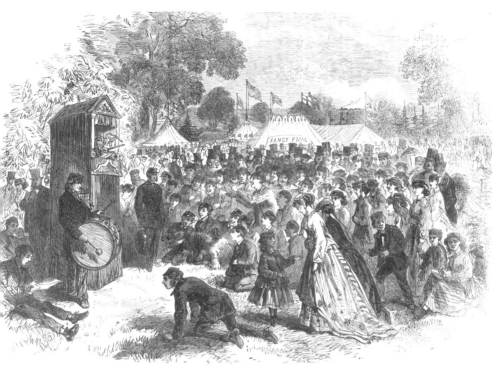

Summer Festival at the Earlswood Asylum for Idiots, Redhill. Illustrated London News, 1867.

building proved to be far too small and a sister institution at Essex Hall near Colchester, Essex was annexed to the National Asylum known as the *Eastern Counties Asylum for Idiots and Imbeciles,* later called the *Royal Eastern Counties Institution.* Both the Highgate and Colchester institutions amalgamated and relocated in 1855 to Redhill in Surrey as the purpose-built *Royal Earlswood Asylum for Idiots.*

Dr John Langdon Down (1828–96), after whom Down's syndrome was named, was medical superintendent at Earlswood until 1868. He published his theory of an ethnic classification of idiots in 1866 referring to Down's as 'the Mongolian type of idiot', hence Mongolism. With his wife, Mary Crellin, Langdon Down founded the Normansfield Training Institution at Teddington in the south of London in 1868, and relocated there. Normansfield was a private, residential facility for idiot and imbecile children of the upper and middle classes. The fees for this exclusive establishment were 150 guineas a year, which was greater than the fees for an English public school at that time. It was originally intended for the education of idiot children but developed into a convenient repository for them. Ironically in 1905, Langdon Brown's son Reginald, who was also a medical practitioner involved in his father's work at Normansfield, had a son, John Langdon, named after his grandfather. John Langdon Down Junior had Down's syndrome.

In 1864, a subscription institution to cater for and educate idiot children in the south-west of England called the *Western Counties Asylum for Idiots* was opened at Star Cross, near Exeter, initially in a house with two acres of land rented from William Courtney, 11th Earl of Devon (1807–88), who was also the asylum's first president. A criterion for admission was that children had to be certified educable, and consequently most patients were imbeciles rather than idiots. By 1870 Star Cross housed forty pupils and an appeal for funds to expand the institution by donation and subscription was launched. In 1877 a new building surrounded by seven acres of grounds was opened. This was able to accommodate sixty boys and forty girls. It was expanded between 1886 and 1909, and by 1913 a total of 1,451 imbeciles and idiots had passed through the institution. In 1914 it became known as the Western Counties Institution certified under the Companies Act as 'a residential special school for mental defectives'.

Also, in 1864, the *Northern Counties Asylum for Idiots and Imbeciles of the seven northern counties* was established at Lancaster, Lancashire, later renamed the *Royal Albert Asylum,* and subsequently, the *Royal Albert Hospital*. It accepted imbecile patients from the seven northern counties of England between the ages of 6 and 15. It was re-opened in 1870 at Ashton Road, Lancaster as an institution for the care and education of idiot, imbecile and weak-minded children. By 1909 there were 662 children in residence.

Dr Bell Fletcher, a physician, and Mr Jonathan Kimball, a surgeon, made financial provision for a charitable 'asylum for twenty idiot girls' which opened in 1866 at Knowle, Solihull in the West Midlands in a house that was originally known as Dorridge Grove Idiot Asylum. It promoted a philosophy of 'happiness and affection, teaching the idiot the use of their senses.' Although Dorridge Grove started as a small-scale establishment, it was very successful. The demand for places led to a new asylum being built in 1872 to provide for the increasing numbers of idiot children of both genders from all over the Midlands of England. This replacement asylum was renamed the *Midland Counties Middle Class Idiots Asylum* and was very much praised by John Bucknill, the Lord

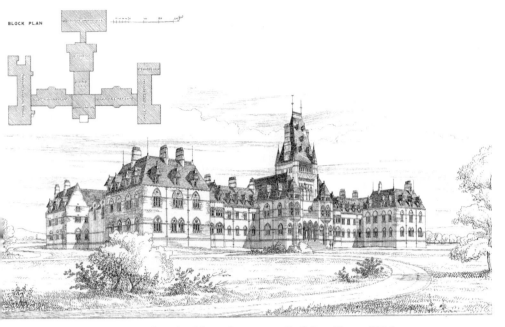

The Royal Albert Asylum for Idiots, Lancaster. Building News, 1874

Chancellor's Visitor in Lunacy, in 1873. Bucknill lamented upon the situation of 'a neglected idiot':

> *The misery of a neglected idiot is an awful thing to contemplate.*
> *He is the most solitary of human beings, cut off from his kind, shut*
> *out by his infirmity from all feeling with his fellow-men – all*
> *sympathy; shut out also from the enjoyment of life, even animal*
> *enjoyment. Often he cannot use sight or hearing so as to*
> *distinguish objects or sounds. Often he cannot walk or stand. Often*
> *he is tortured with painful bodily infirmities. In a private house he*
> *is often an intolerable burden, an incubus, a waking nightmare.*

There was a general consensus at that time that mentally impaired children were better cared for in institutions which could cater for their specific needs rather than being looked after by their own families at home – where they were usually neglected and hidden out of sight and out of mind. Nevertheless, at that time, there was less social stigma to having a child who was mentally disabled at birth or shortly afterwards than having a member of the family who became mentally deranged in

173

adolescence or adulthood. This situation was particularly felt by upper and middle class families who sent their mentally handicapped offspring to Normansfield and remained proud of the progress their children made. For the working classes however, a child with a disability of any type was a drain on the resources of the family and these children were generally not treated with such pride and care – many were regularly neglected. For some the poorhouse or the asylum was a better option for their overall welfare than remaining in the family home.

However, it was not always the case that upper and middle class families took a pride in the abilities of their mentally impaired offspring. For some 'out of sight and out of mind' was still an important consideration.

In England and Wales the *Idiots Act* of 1886 was the first Act to provide for mental disability as a separate entity from mental illness. It was intended to provide a framework for the admission, supervision, education, and training, for idiots and imbeciles. A Royal Commission on the Care and Control of the Feeble-Minded was set up in 1904 with a warrant 'to consider the existing methods of dealing with idiots and epileptics, and with imbecile, feeble-minded, or defective-persons' not certified under the Lunacy Laws.

The *Mental Deficiency Act,* 1913 repealed the former Act.

- 'Idiots' were now defined as 'those so deeply defective as to be unable to guard themselves against common physical dangers';
- 'Imbeciles' were those 'whose defectiveness does not amount to idiocy, but is so pronounced that they are not capable of managing themselves or their affairs, or, in the case of children, of being taught to do so';
- 'Feeble-minded persons' were those 'whose weakness does not amount to imbecility, yet who require care, supervision, or control, for their protection or for the protection of others, or, in the case of children, are incapable of receiving benefit from the instruction in ordinary schools'; and,
- 'Moral imbeciles' were those 'displaying mental weakness coupled with strong dangerous, and criminal dispositions, on whom punishment would have little or no detrimental effect'.

The 1913 Act placed closer regulation on the identification and institutionalisation of children with learning disabilities. It proposed taking them out of Poor Law institutions and prisons, and placing them into newly established colonies.

Case study: John Lucas

In June 1879, an 11-year-old boy was admitted to Denbighshire Asylum in Wales. Despite his love for burning things he took most pleasure from being lifted up in the air, which made him laugh with joy. John William Guy Lucas was the eldest son of Thomas Pennington Lucas, a medical practitioner, and his wife Mary Frances Sarah, née Davies. The couple had four children following their marriage at St Margaret's, Westminster in 1868. Thomas Lucas was the son of a Wesleyan minister and Mary Davies was the daughter of a surgeon. Despite their good education and family background, their eldest child was classified as an idiot – a condition the asylum authorities stressed was hereditary as his paternal grandfather was in Northampton Asylum at the same time.

Despite both his father and son being in asylum care, one as a private patient the other as a pauper, and his wife having died, Thomas Lucas emigrated to Australia for health reasons and did not return. His three younger children eventually joined him and he re-married and started a new family. His eldest child remained a pauper patient in Denbigh asylum until he died from epilepsy on 15 April 1889.

In Scotland, the Baldovan Institution, situated about three miles from Dundee, was founded in 1852 as an orphanage and school for imbecile and idiot children through the generosity of Sir John Ogilvie, Baronet, of Baldovan (1803–90) and his wife Jane, Lady Ogilvie (d. 1861). Their own son had a learning disability and attended the pioneering residential school for cretins established by Dr Johann Jakob Guggenbühl (1816–63) on the Abendberg, above Interlachen, Switzerland in 1842. Other voluntary contributions to Baldovan included a donation of £100 from its patrons, Queen Victoria and Prince Albert. The orphanage opened in November 1854 to provide accommodation for thirty girls, and the separate asylum in January 1855 to house a further ten children who had to be under the age of 10 years on admission and be expected to remain in the asylum for five years. In 1856 the Institution changed its name to *The Baldovan*

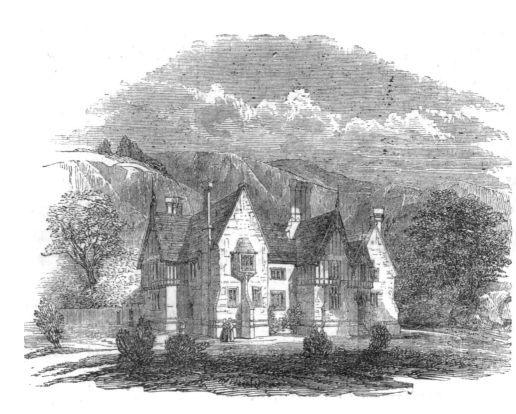

Orphanage and Asylum for Idiot Children at Baldovan near Dundee. Illustrated London News, 1863.

Asylum for Imbecile Children. The orphanage moved out in 1867 and the asylum specialised in the care of idiot and imbecile children. By 1879 the asylum cared for seventy children, and by 1904 this number had increased to 160. By 1915 Baldovan had 229 resident children.

The 1857 Royal Commission on Lunacy in Scotland reported that of the 7,400 lunatics in that country, 2,600 were congenital idiots and imbeciles. Although the ensuing *Lunacy (Scotland) Act* of 1857 made no provision for children, the Scottish Lunacy Board's first annual report recorded and highlighted the work of the 'Idiot Schools' at Baldovan and another institute specifically for idiot and imbecile children at Gayfield Square, Edinburgh. Mention was made of the on-going efforts to raise funds for a model national institution in Scotland. These efforts were advanced by the Society for Education of Imbecile Youth in Scotland established in 1859. Rather than raising funds by relying on a few large donations, the idea of a penny subscription was introduced. Sufficient funds snowballed to allow the board of directors to purchase land. As this was to be the national institution, the Stenhouse Estate near Larbert was chosen because of its geographical location right in the centre of Scotland, and its network of rail links. The Board commissioned Frederick Pilkington (1832–98), a Scottish architect practising in the Victorian High Gothic revival style, to design the school.

Dr David Brodie was appointed the first medical superintendent of The Scottish National Institute for the Education of Imbecile Children at Larbert, near Falkirk, Stirlingshire in 1862. He had previously supervised the Edinburgh Idiot Asylum, a 'home and school', which he founded with his wife in the autumn of 1855 in Gayfield Square, Edinburgh. The children from Edinburgh were transferred to the Scottish National Institute when it opened in May 1863. It was initially intended to provide accommodation for children between the ages of 6 and 12, although older and younger children could be admitted on merit. There were three categories of admission:

- Private pupils were charged at a standard rate of £50 p.a.; with a reduced rate of between £25 to £40 p.a. for families who were not paupers but could prove that they could not afford the full rate; (There was also a higher rate of up to £150 per annum for high-dependency children with specific or special needs, or who needed extra care and attendant(s));
- Elected pupils (elected through the annual ballot of the subscribers to the Institution and so admitted without charge, to stay for a maximum of five years);
- Paupers, whose maintenance was paid for by Parish poor law funds through their Parochial Boards.

Those paying a subscription or donation were given voting rights in proportion to their contribution – 10s gave 1 vote; £1 gave 2 votes and so on. Both Baldovan and the Scottish National Institute had a range of criteria for admission and rejected children who appeared incurable or were purely epileptic. The educational agenda was promoted for both institutions. The 1863 prospectus stated:

The education proposed will include not only the simple elements of instruction usually taught in common schools, where that is

*possible, but will embrace a course of training in the more
practical matters of everyday life – the cultivation of habits of
cleanliness, propriety, self-management, self-reliance, and the
development and enlargement of a capacity of useful occupation.*

In 1887 there were forty-three patients at the Scottish National Institute,
rising to ninety-five in 1870.

In a typical year, 1889, there were forty-two new admissions to the
Scottish National Institute at Larbert: twenty-one boys with an age range
from 7 to 15 years; and twenty-one girls with an age range from 6 to 14
years. By 1906 there were 296 children resident in the Institution, and by
1914 almost 400. Most children were discharged from Baldovan or the
Scottish National Institute when they reached their mid-teens. Some
returned to their communities able to do simple work to support
themselves. A very few were given menial employment in the institutions
in which they spent their teenage years, such as messengers or ward
attendants. However, despite the good intentions of Baldovan and the
Scottish National Institute to educate and train imbeciles, the majority of
patients with learning disabilities on reaching adulthood were admitted
to district asylums or poorhouses.

Most childhood 'idiots', as they aged, progressed into the asylum
system as adult idiots.

Consanguinity, otherwise derogatorily called inbreeding, had long
been considered one of the causes of congenital mental impairment.

Dr W.A.F. Browne, as Inspector of Lunacy, when visiting the Hallcross
Madhouse in Musselburgh, Midlothian in 1860 stumbled across seven
siblings, all belonging to the same family and all considered to be idiots.
He remarked:

*In passing through I saw five old and apparently aged men, seated
together around a table and apart from the other patients. They
smiled and spoke a few words; garbled or jargonised. My
companion said 'they liked to dine together.' On complimenting
him for his attention to their wishes, he answered, 'Oh they are all
brothers.' On going to the Department for females I observed two
quiet, elderly women indulged in the same way – 'these' said my
guide 'are sisters, and sisters of the five brothers.' They were the
children of poor, but industrious and self-supporting parents who*

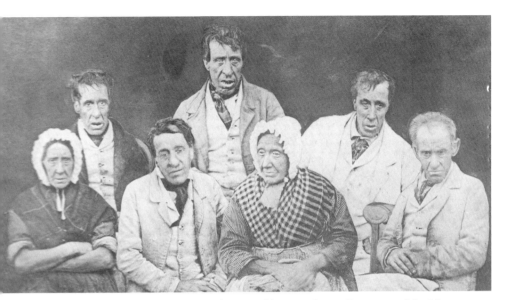

The Wightman family from Humbie, Haddingtonshire. Courtesy of Lothian Health Services Archive, Edinburgh University Library.

were somewhat eccentric; and believed to be Cousins, or related. – They are all, in different degrees, imbecile; ineducable; irresponsible and incapable of guiding or maintaining themselves.

This was clearly a family with inherited mental incapacity.

Dr W.A.F. Browne noted that Mungo Wightman (47) was solitary, taciturn and worked laboriously in the garden; Thomas Wightman (51) was occasionally violent; William Wightman (53) would not wash and could not speak intelligibly; David Wightman (56) was passionately fond of washing stockings, but would not work outdoors; Helen Wightman (65) was affectionate, attentive, tractable and neat in dress; James Wightman (69) was childish, confused and excitable, and did nothing; Agnes Wightman (71) was quiet and inoffensive but spoke indistinctly.

The siblings were from a family of twelve children – eight of whom had impaired mental faculties. Born and brought up in Humbie, East Lothian, Scotland, the Wightmans' care fell to their parish on the death of their parents John Wightman and Elizabeth Pendrich after 1841. Another sister, Elizabeth, married and had her own family and she cared for the sister closest in age to herself, Isabella, who was classified an imbecile. This home care saved Isabella from entering the asylum or poorhouse.

Case study: Oliver Twist

Admission note for Oliver Twist, 1868. Montrose Royal Asylum case notes. Courtesy of Dundee University Archive Services.

In September 1868 the police in Aberdeen, Edinburgh and Glasgow were wired informing them of the escape of a lunatic from Aberdeen Royal Asylum. An Edinburgh policeman spotted 'a glaikit looking fellow, obviously insane, who was unable to give any account of himself' and assuming him to be the escapee, 'at once took him to Aberdeen'. However, on his arrival at the asylum there, the officer was informed that this was not the escaped man and therefore he took him back to Edinburgh and 'set him adrift'.

Later that day the mistaken lunatic was found at Gorebridge Railway Station 'making the most horrible faces at a train as it went by.' He was arrested and subsequently sent to Edinburgh Royal Asylum on a sheriff's warrant. He was a deaf-mute and could give no account of his name or origins. The staff dubbed him 'Oliver Twist' and the admission records state 'he has evidently been thoroughly trained in an Idiot institution.'

Unable to read or write, he gesticulated with his hands and was able to make guttural noises from his throat, but could not articulate in any other way. On the 6 November 1868 he was transferred to Montrose Royal Asylum. He worked well on the asylum farm, but he was 'prone to interfere with the other patients and consequently was frequently hit by them.' The Montrose clinical records stop in 1882. The Register of Discharges and Removals show that 'Oliver Twist' was 'relieved' to Stonehaven Combination Poorhouse on 2 July 1885 and the 1891 Census shows him resident there, age stated as 55 years, and his occupation given as a seaman, place of birth unknown. 'Oliver' died in the poorhouse on 14 May 1893, aged 56 years from phthisis pulmonalis (tuberculosis of the lungs) of a year's duration – presumably acquired in the poorhouse. His actual identity remains an enigma.

A private Institute for the Training, Education and Maintenance of Idiotic and Imbecile Children was founded in 1868 at Lucan Spa, County Dublin, by Dr Henry Hutchison Stewart. The Stewart Institute for Idiots was 'based on Protestant principles of the broadest and unsectarian character.' To emphasise its educational aspirations, the children were called 'pupils' rather than patients. By 1875, the Stewart Institution was overcrowded and the management committee purchased the mansion and lands of the late Lord Donoghmore at Palmerstown, five miles west of Dublin. The premises were converted and extended and in 1879 all the pupils of the Lucan Institution were transferred there. In time the name changed to Stewart's Hospital and for almost fifty years, it was the only special provision for mentally handicapped children and adults in all Ireland.

Chapter 14

Epilepsy

The nineteenth century saw progress in the medical understanding of epilepsy – a condition that was always considered to have sinister connotations. From the beginning of written history an awareness of epilepsy existed, and a variety of myths, medical explanations and mystique surrounded what, in ancient times, had been described as a 'Sacred Disease'. A full understanding of epilepsy by the nineteenth century, whilst very much in its infancy, advanced greatly due to the invaluable contribution of pioneering medical practitioners.

In the ancient world, it was believed that gods were responsible for epileptic fits, with the body and soul overcome by a demon or spirit. The biblical references to epilepsy in the synoptic gospels showed Jesus removing 'foul spirits' and rebuking them. This powerful image would have been known throughout the Christian world and, as a result, made the epileptic a person to be feared and shunned by society. In the astrological literature of pagan antiquity there was a widespread association between epilepsy and the moon making those afflicted with the disorder 'lunatics', from the Greek *luna* meaning moon. These beliefs were difficult to disprove without the technology of modern medical science and there was much speculation as to the causes and cure of those 'possessed by the devil'.

Some physicians also believed that epilepsy could be caused by witchcraft. *The Malleus Maleficarum* (The Hammer of Witches) written by Kramer and Sprenger in 1487 was a classical textbook that reported cases of epilepsy inflicted 'by means of eggs which have been buried with dead bodies, especially the dead bodies of witches'. It was believed that every type of disease could be caused by witchcraft and epilepsy was no exception.

The witchcraft craze that took place in Renaissance Europe extended to the New World with the Salem Witch Trials of the 1690s, which resulted in women who suffered from hysteria or epilepsy becoming easy targets. These two illnesses were most frequently confused with witchcraft or demonic possession, particularly if accompanied by tremors, convulsions or altered consciousness. In some parts of the world superstition and witchcraft continue to be blamed for epilepsy. By the nineteenth century in Europe, however, medical explanations were being put forward and the causes of the disorder began to be better understood. Several eminent physicians and alienists attempted to define the causes of epilepsy in the nineteenth century but many were unable to agree to its actual causation. Jean Étienne Dominique Esquirol (1772–1840), an alienist and epileptologist in Paris, was reluctant to believe its cause stemmed from the brain but other physicians, in particular John Hughlings Jackson (1835–1911), recognised that this was its cause. He advanced this aetiology more than any other doctor and worked from The National Hospital for Neurology and Neurosurgery in Queen Square, London – which has been described as the 'cradle of British Neurology'.

During the 1880s, the *British Medical Journal* observed and recorded the lack of facilities for non-insane epileptics, despite there being provision for those classed as 'epileptic and insane' or 'epileptic and imbecile' in the asylum system. However, at the same time an editorial comment in *The Lancet*, referring to epileptics as 'poor people', suggested that they should be kept together for reasons of safety. It was clear in the mind not only of medical professionals, but also writers at this time, that epilepsy was better not seen, and was something to be feared. It is also interesting to observe from the above two articles that an asylum was clearly considered an appropriate place for epileptics, regardless of mental capacity or social class.

A diagnosis of epilepsy extends beyond the physical and biological impact on the body and brain of an individual and also affects the economic, psychological and social aspects of life. This impact would have been all the greater during the nineteenth century when medication was limited and the prospects for individuals with uncontrolled epilepsy were bleak. In 1857, Sir Charles Locock (1799–1875) discovered the anticonvulsant and sedative qualities of potassium bromide and it became regularly used to treat epileptic seizures and nervous disorders until the discovery of phenobarbital in 1912.

The prognosis for patients with any form of epilepsy was not favourable and many became long-term patients who died in asylums;

the disorder was widely regarded as incurable by nineteenth century doctors.

Epileptic patients were occasionally admitted to asylums hoping for a cure, but generally because they were no longer able to be cared for within the home or workhouse. Asylum admission records often described these patients as 'dangerous', but studies have shown that many only became so during, or prior to, a seizure. Many of the asylums built in the latter half of the nineteenth century followed the recommendations of Dr W.A.F. Browne, medical superintendent of the Crichton Royal Institute, Dumfries between 1838 and 1857 and a Commissioner in Lunacy for Scotland 1857–70. Browne believed that asylums should be built as palaces with extensive grounds for the therapeutic care of the afflicted. There is evidence from asylum case notes that following the changes to the asylum system in the latter half of the nineteenth century, the asylum was a better option for many epileptic patients than the workhouse. For those unable to pay for private asylum care, the county asylum was an appealing alternative particularly if the asylum had purpose built provision for epileptic patients.

A home specifically for epileptics was founded in Maghull, Liverpool, in 1888. The home, which was registered as a charity, was originally purchased following a generous donation from a Liverpool gentleman. In 1892 the Honorary Secretary of the charity committee, William Grisewood, made an appeal to the people of Liverpool for financial assistance in building additional accommodation. He provided a description of the home and the benefits to its patients:

> *The home is an old manor house, with lawns, plantations, gardens, orchard and even a moat. It has been made to accommodate about 48 patients. The charges range from 7s. 6d. to £2. 2s. per week according to accommodation.*
>
> *The medical treatment of the patients is carefully attended to by the honorary medical staff, and a well-trained matron and nurses have been provided and are gradually increased in number as occasion requires. The gardens and grounds furnish outdoor work for the male patients, housework and needlework occupy the females. Kindness and consideration for each other are strongly inculcated. Their friends are always welcome when they call to see them and frequent entertainments are provided.*

This home remains today in Maghull as the Parkhaven Trust and continues to provide a caring environment.

In 1892 The National Society for the Employment of Epileptics (NSEE) was launched by a group of London philanthropists and medical men. The aim of the society was to provide suitable accommodation for epileptics who were able to work but were unable to find suitable employment due to their medical condition. Skippings Farm near Chalfont St Peter in Buckinghamshire was bought by the society and the first patients were admitted in 1894. Initially the 'colonists' were men of 'reasonable behaviour and mental ability'. They were charged 10s a week, although financial help was provided by way of an annuity fund for those who could not afford the full amount. The original staff consisted of a lady superintendent, a bailiff, a male attendant, a nurse and a female servant. The 'colonists' worked on the land or within the building six days a week and were visited on a regular basis by doctors from The National Hospital in London.

Additional epileptic colonies were built following the success of Chalfont St Peter and by 1900 there were seven permanent homes there accommodating ninety men and over forty women. As in asylums however, men and women were strictly segregated. From 1909, children were admitted to the colony when the local school authority funded the building of two additional homes and a school. An epileptic colony specifically for children, 'The Lingfield Epileptic Colony', was built in Crowborough in Sussex at the end of the nineteenth century and potassium bromide was given to selected children to determine its usefulness in curing their disorder.

An epileptic colony called the 'Colony of Mercy' was founded in Kilmacolm, Renfrewshire, Scotland in the early 1900s. The founder was philanthropist William Quarrier who had also established a series of orphan homes to remove poor children from the streets and into clean country air. The 'Colony of Mercy' initially provided care for epileptic women and children. It had a workshop to keep them employed when the weather was unsuitable for them to be outside. This was very much in keeping with the philosophy of Chalfont St Peter, which also believed that epileptics should be encouraged to work when they could. These epilepsy centres continue to this day.

However, despite the success of epileptic colonies many epileptic patients had no choice but to be admitted to asylums or workhouses when their condition became unmanageable at home. Many epileptics remained within their communities if seizures were slight, or they had a solid support network and were able to work. For those who did not however, a workhouse or asylum was their only choice.

There were six main reasons why an individual with epilepsy would seek assistance:

- An increase in seizures which required medical assistance;
- Dangerous or aggressive behaviour that put others at risk;
- Threats of suicide;
- Lack of support from family or friends;
- An inability to remain within employment;
- The belief that they could be cured with appropriate medical treatment.

Following changes to the asylum system in the nineteenth century, and new purpose built asylums, provision for epileptic patients improved. Those admitted had access to medical help and a range of experimental 'medication' that was aimed to reduce seizures. Some asylums had special wards for epileptics where additional care had been taken to provide padding to fireguards and other furniture in case of seizures. The asylum at Macclesfield in Cheshire provided wider, padded pews at the rear of their purpose-built church specifically for the use of epileptic patients.

The Glamorgan County Asylum in Bridgend installed a machine that they called a 'tell-tale' clock. This acted as a complete and infallible check on the night-nurse and attendants in the observation dormitories set aside for epileptic and suicidal cases. A cylinder with a printed form placed around it was housed in a small case beneath the face of the clock. Wires connected the clock with the observation dormitories, and the attendants were required to communicate with the office every quarter of an hour. By touching a small button, a brass pin in the clock made a mark on the paper around the cylinder, which allowed the medical superintendent to check whether the attendants had remained vigilant through the night. This was deemed both a necessary precaution and a satisfactory method of ensuring the safety of epileptic and suicidal patients.

It was recognised that epilepsy was not curable and additional comfort was attempted. The presence of a dog called Mab on the epileptic ward at the Macclesfield Asylum helped provide a more homelike atmosphere for many patients, the majority of whom would never recover.

During a study of female patients admitted to Parkside Asylum in Cheshire between 1871 and 1901, it was noted that nearly eighty per cent of female epileptic admissions were unmarried women. The stigma attached to epilepsy was high in the nineteenth century – the social consequences of marriage to an epileptic, and the possibility of children being left without a mother because of asylum admission, would have been a difficult choice for many men to make. Children were strongly dependent on the presence of both parents within the family home. With the father as the breadwinner, often working long hours, it was the responsibility of the mother to care for the children and organise household affairs – also often combined with earning a wage to supplement the family income. The absence of either parent from the home often made it difficult for families to remain together for economic reasons, and many families were forced to split to ensure their survival.

Case study: Bridget Kelly
Bridget Kelly was admitted to an asylum on four occasions during the 1880s. Her daughter Mary, despite also having epilepsy and defined as an imbecile, spent time in the workhouse while her mother was absent from home. It is possible Mary's father, Patrick Kelly, was unable to care on his own for a child with complex difficulties when his wife was admitted to the asylum and was obliged to have her cared for within the workhouse system.

Case study: Margaret Broadhurst
Described as 'not mentally impaired' but 'dull and slow of mind', Margaret Broadhurst had two small children when she was admitted to Parkside on 30 March 1882. However, her asylum case notes make no mention of them. Margaret suffered from severe epileptic fits and frequent bouts of acute mania that prevented her from working. It is also likely that these conditions prevented her from caring adequately for her young children. Although merely conjecture it is possible that in order to keep both her and her children safe, her husband made the decision to request her admission to Parkside.

Children born with disabilities were similarly a problem within the nineteenth century household, particularly if both parents worked and relied on their children to help contribute to the family income. Epileptic children would be an extra burden and one that would require many families to make a painful choice.

Case study: Mary Jane Percival

Mary Jane was only 10 years old when she was admitted to Parkside Asylum in Macclesfield, Cheshire from Knutsford Workhouse in 1890. Diagnosed with 'Imbecility and Epilepsy' she was described as a quick-witted child, good at evading questions she did not wish to answer about her mischievous behaviour. The workhouse staff commented that Mary Jane continually asked to taste the poisons in the workhouse surgery and needed to be continually monitored. It was this fascination with medicine that resulted in her move from the workhouse into the asylum and she was admitted onto the epilepsy ward.

Mary Jane knew where she was when admitted to Parkside and could recall the names of her parents and siblings. The medical superintendent there commented that Mary Jane had 'been left pretty much to the freedom of her own will' and as a result 'is flippant and forward in her manner'. Mary Jane provided answers to questions when it suited her, and clearly knew where she was and was not distressed about it. The medical officer observed that she was 'a poor delicate looking creature but able to run about and enjoy herself in the grounds.' One of the more sensible patients was given charge of her and her behaviour improved very rapidly.

Mary Jane had multiple seizures. In the early days following admission these amounted to a twitching of the left eyelid and the drawing up of her left arm. Going pale after they had ceased, the case notes described her as 'stupid and drowsy' for a few minutes afterwards. Mary Jane became accustomed to feigning seizures – what would now be termed 'pseudo-seizures' – but when the nurse pointed these out to her they stopped. However, she had an average of two genuine epileptiform seizures each day during which she lost consciousness.

By May 1891 her fits had become extremely frequent, with often twenty each night. The medical officer noted that she looked distraught and prescribed chloral hydrate and potassium bromide. Belladonna was also tried. The medication had little to no effect and the medical officers determined that the increase in seizures was due to the onset of menstruation.

In February 1902 Mary Jane became unwell with an increased temperature and was put to bed; she was later moved to a different ward and monitored. There are no reports of seizures during this period, however she deteriorated rapidly, became very weak and was given several hypodermics of brandy. She died later the same evening and a post mortem revealed she had phthisis pulmonalis – a form of tuberculosis. She was only 21 years old.

Mary Jane's younger brother, Robert John, was also admitted to the same asylum on 8 July 1898 categorised as an 'idiot with epilepsy'. He was 7 years old. He was incapable of speech, bit and beat himself, and clung onto anyone near him in a distressed way. No mention is made in his case notes of the death of his parents in 1901 and 1905.

His presence in the asylum is not mentioned in Mary Jane's case notes and, due to their difference in age and the length of time she had been in Parkside, she may never have met him. Robert John died on 27 June 1915 in Parkside Asylum.

Chapter 15

General Paralysis of the Insane

As I was a-walking by the banks o' the Ugie,
Come, my dear friends, and this story I'll relate:
I spied a dear comrade all dressed in white flannel,
Dressed in white flannel and cruel was his fate.

[CHORUS] Oh the mercury was beating, the limestone was reeking,
His tongue all in flames hung over his chin.
A hole in his bosom, his teeth were a-closing.
Bad luck to the girlie that gied him the glim.

And had she but told me, oh when she dishonoured me;
Had she but told me of it in time –
I might have been cured by those pills of white mercury,
Now I'm a young man cut down in my prime.

My parents, they warned me and oft times they chided,
With those young flash girls do not sport and play.
I never listened, no, I never heeded,
I just carried on in my own wicked way.

It's down on the corner two flash girls were talking;
One to the other did whisper and say
"There goes that young man who once was so jolly,
Now for his sins his poor body must pay".

Oh doctor, dear doctor, before your departure,
Take all these bottles of mercury away.
Send for the minister to say a prayer over me,
So they can lay my poor body in the clay

– Traditional folk song,
Aberdeenshire (Scotland)

General Paralysis of the Insane (GPI), which was also called 'general paresis' or 'paralytic dementia', was a devastating and rapidly progressive type of insanity. It was a neurological disease prevalent in the nineteenth and early twentieth centuries that killed many people. Victims were mainly in early middle-age, most often in their early forties. It was caused by end-stage syphilis – yet the link between that particular venereal disease and GPI was not formally established until the 1920s.

In the nineteenth century, GPI was considered to be a physical and behavioural manifestation of an organic brain disease. It was viewed as a 'form of insanity complicated by paralysis' rather than a 'form of paralysis complicated by insanity'. Post mortem examinations in Paris during the 1820s demonstrated remarkable physical changes in the brains of insane patients who had been diagnosed with *paralysie générale*. This linked the physical symptoms of GPI to organic brain disease. GPI was a slow and silent killer with the psychiatric symptoms first appearing many years after first bodily infection – in some cases as long as thirty years later.

The physical symptoms of GPI included shooting or burning muscle pains, progressive muscle weakness, impaired speech with a weak or tremulous voice and trembling tongue, generalised shaking, visual impairment as a result of unequal pupils, poor balance and a loss of control of the limbs. The loss of control of a sufferer's arms caused exaggerated shaking of the hands so that they could not drink from a cup without spilling its contents, and loss of control of their legs made them unsteady on their feet, usually with the patient falling forwards when attempting to walk. The progression of the illness could lead to convulsions and eventually to a complete loss of function. The prognosis of GPI was bleak and always fatal. Death could occur from gradual exhaustion, convulsions, brain haemorrhage, or by choking or the inhalation of vomit if the swallowing reflex was lost.

The mental symptoms were often dramatic with intense euphoria, and always included delusions, hallucinations, lack of insight, irritability, mood changes, memory loss and inappropriate behaviour. Disinhibition and spending large sums of money were common manifestations of the behavioural digressions. The delusions were typically those of grandeur in terms of wealth, strength, self-importance, social-importance, ambition or relationships. Many sufferers ran into financial and legal difficulties because of their erratic behaviour.

The actual cause of GPI was much debated in medical circles

throughout the nineteenth century when most doctors believed that syphilis could be just one of the many and various causes. Other aetiologies put forward included 'general debauchery' – sexual excesses and heavy alcohol or tobacco consumption; 'adverse circumstances' (particularly for males) or 'domestic trouble' (for females); over-work or over-study; bereavement; a 'kick from a horse'; and, heredity. Sufferers may have demonstrated more than one of these 'causes'. As many sufferers were married, employed, educated and 'respectable' middle-class men, there was a huge Victorian reluctance to link GPI exclusively with syphilis.

Four to five times as many men as women were admitted to asylums in the nineteenth century with a diagnosis of GPI. The prevalence was comparatively low in rural areas, but in cities the rates were much higher and by 1902, a staggering twenty-one per cent of male admissions to the Royal Edinburgh Asylum were said to be general paralytics, and thirty-four per cent of deaths were attributed to GPI. In 1904 the total number of deaths from GPI in Scottish asylums was said to be 1,795 with approximately 2,250 deaths from GPI in England and Wales in that year.

In terms of treatment, even after the link between GPI and syphilis had been confirmed, there was no effective therapeutic remedy until the use of penicillin in the 1940s. Up until that point, the reality was that, once given a diagnosis of GPI, a patient was deemed to be incurable and doomed to die. Sir Thomas Clouston, Medical Superintendent of the Royal Edinburgh Asylum described GPI in 1876 as 'one absolutely hopeless disease … which, once being recognised, the patient's doom is held to be sealed, without a chance of respite … the most deadly disease of asylumdom.'

In the nineteenth century, mercury pastes were used topically to treat the primary syphilitic sores known as 'chancres' obtained after first contact in the early stages of the disease. Many believed that it worked, despite inducing nausea and pain. Medication in the form of 'pills of white mercury' was administered as an oral therapy for syphilis in the mid-nineteenth century. The dose required to effect a 'cure' was quite toxic and led to excessive uncontrollable salivation and profuse sweating.

In GPI, palliative care was provided by way of tender nursing care and by the use of sedatives to calm and sedate the patients during their terminal illness. Complete rest was considered necessary. Drugs used included paraldehyde, sulphonal, calomel, chloral hydrate, hyoscine and potassium bromides, or a combination of some or all of these. Complete rest and good nursing became the mainstay of therapy. The intensive nursing required for these incurable cases took up a disproportionate amount of limited asylum resources. Particular attention was paid to the prevention of pressure sores (bed sores) and waterbeds were in use in the 1890s for bedridden patients.

Many other chemical therapies were experimented with after the failure of oral mercury. Bismuth replaced mercury from the 1880s often administered by intramuscular injection. Iodides, usually of potassium but also sulphur or ammonium, were used to treat syphilis. They had side effects of a dry cough and skin rashes. Treatment with arsenic was tried later (in the form of salvarsan and tryparsamide). In the early 1920s treatment was attempted by inoculating patients with malaria to induce a therapeutic fever. The first definitive laboratory test for syphilis, the Wassermann reaction, was developed in 1906 to detect syphilis in the blood or cerebrospinal fluid. After the discovery of penicillin in 1928, GPI became treatable and curable.

Clouston issued guidelines to his medical officers for taking case notes of paralytic patients on their admission to the asylum.

HISTORY
Inquire carefully into the history of the case for facts which may throw light on the nature of the malady. Disposition – Enquire whether eccentric, gloomy, cheerful or keen. Hereditary history – other diseases: Enquire for Hysteria, Fits, Paralysis, St Vitus' Dance, Eccentricity, Marked Depravity, etc. Also for Phthisis (Decline), Apoplexy, Heart Disease, etc.

STATE ON ADMISSION
Observe whether there be anything in the emotional state, or in the nature of the delusions to indicate special treatment. Memory – old events, recent events, permanent facts. Pupils – shape, size, reaction to light. Nervous system – under this heading look for signs of paralysis in the motor area, including defects of speech, also test for muscular power and gait; and make any notes concerning organic reflexes. Other abnormalities – look carefully for surface markings of all sorts. Lungs – note cough, if any, and

nature of sputum. Palate – three varieties: 1. Average – broad and low; 2. Nervous – high but well-shaped; 3. Deformed. Pulse – test the pulse with reference to size, rate, rhythm (regularity) and tension (compressibility).

Case studies: delusions of grandeur

Robert Murdoch, a 46-year-old married sailor, believed he was the commander of the largest ship in the world. He thought that he was one of the strongest men on Earth. If he whistled, a million men would come at once to his aid.

Janet Scott, an unmarried 27-year-old seamstress from Hawick, believed herself to be an extremely important person who possessed a considerable amount of properties throughout the Scottish Borders.

Alban Cottrill, a 37-year-old unmarried silk-weaver from Macclesfield, believed that he could do almost anything because he was a great doctor of divinity of the Catholic unity and was the deputy of one of the Saints of his church. Alban was going to purchase the largest library in the world for £4.

Albert Sidebottom, a 40-year-old unmarried railway clerk, had delusions with regard to property and marriage. He boasted of purchasing horses, buildings, phaetons and of ordering 'lots of goods'.

Francis Kyle Richardson thought that he possessed huge sums of money, was the owner of great estates, and was enormously strong. He believed he was a 'very important man and will set things right in this asylum.'

Anthony Sloane, a 33-year-old married grocer from Dukinfield, thought that he had hundreds of thousands of pounds owing to him and that he was forsaken of God for not attending to his religious duties. He stated that he was 'a low high man not a high low one.'

Case study: William Anderson

In 1871, William Anderson appeared to be an intelligent, married man with a good respectable job. To the outside world he was a pillar of society – he was employed as a coach trimmer earning over £2 a week and was a member of the Baptist Church in Congleton, Cheshire. His asylum records note that he was a native of Fife, Scotland. But William had a past that began to catch up with him that year. His behaviour changed rapidly, he spent money recklessly and became confused, loquacious, and excited in mood with wandering ideas. William became violent and abusive towards his wife, Ann. He was admitted to Parkside Asylum in Cheshire on 1 June 1871 where he talked about his delusions of having been a mercenary in the American Civil War. William had a shaky tongue and twitchy face and was unsteady on his feet. He boasted of his marvellous and grandiose furniture inventions, and that he was going to London to fit up a drawing room for Queen Victoria. William was diagnosed with General Paralysis of the Insane. He was prescribed a variety of medication including chloral hydrate, potassium bromide, and his favourite – a tincture of Indian cannabis – which he declared made him feel much better. He attempted to escape from the asylum by jumping through a window he had broken, and landed on both feet, completely unharmed. William's disease progressed rapidly and he was dead within a year.

Case study: George Logan

The case of George Brown Logan highlights the difficulties in the years before any laboratory testing – the diagnosis of GPI proved so problematic in the nineteenth century that it often could not be made until after death with a post mortem examination confirming or refuting the identification of the disease. The mental symptoms of GPI could easily be confused with other disorders such as mania or acute dementia.

In 1896 George Logan was 30 years old, married, and a master carter. In October that year he travelled from Galashiels in the Scottish Borders to Edinburgh to buy a horse, but instead, he abducted a tramway trace horse. He rode the horse about the streets of Edinburgh in a reckless and erratic manner and was promptly arrested. He was admitted to Edinburgh Royal Asylum and then transferred to Roxburgh District Asylum five days later. The admission diagnosis was 'acute mania' but GPI was also suspected. Physical examination revealed some slurring of speech and a few days later he displayed unequal pupils, but there was not sufficient evidence to substantiate a diagnosis of GPI. George behaved well during his admission and was allowed to leave the asylum to return to his wife and son in January 1897 on six months' probation. The application made by the asylum superintendent to the General Board of Lunacy stated 'although he shows a certain amount of enfeeblement and silliness, he behaves in a quiet and inoffensive manner, employs himself usefully and attends to his own wants.'

George was re-admitted to Borders District Asylum in April 1898 however, when he was voicing delusions that he was missing his arms and head. He displayed slurred speech, a tremulous tongue, shaking hands, a lack of coordination, and weakness of his legs. George's condition gradually and slowly deteriorated and he died in the asylum on 24 January 1901, aged 34, leaving a 4-year-old son. The diagnosis of GPI was confirmed by post mortem examination.

Case Study: Fanny Proudlove
Fanny Proudlove, a 35-year-old unmarried farmhouse servant from Hassall Green in Cheshire, was admitted to Parkside Asylum on 3 March 1886 with a diagnosis of paralytic dementia. She had suffered a paralytic stroke two years previously and was in poor general health. She displayed muscle weakness on the left side of her face and walked on her toes because she was unable to place her feet flat on the ground. Fanny appeared childish in manner and chuckled away to herself. Her speech was incoherent. The medical officer described her as 'a very miserable case of paralytic dementia – incapable of concentration, dirty in her habits and of unhealthy appearance.' Fanny died in the asylum on 15 October 1886 with the cause of death, confirmed by post mortem, being certified as General Paralysis and Acute Pneumonia.

GPI was, in its day, a uniformly fatal disease. A considerable number of people, often married with young families, died in their prime. The social consequences of these deaths were profound.

Chapter 16

Puerperal Insanity

In November 1817, 21-year-old Princess Charlotte, grand-daughter of George III and the only child of George, Prince of Wales, later George IV, gave birth to a stillborn son following a prolonged labour. Despite being under the care of the Royal Obstetrician, Sir Richard Croft (1762–1818), the Princess bled to death. As well as shocking the nation, her death in childbirth undoubtedly increased anxiety for mothers-to-be. Three months later, Sir Richard Croft committed suicide by shooting himself in the head, unable to live with the resulting criticism and the knowledge that he had been responsible for two deaths.

In the nineteenth century many women were anxious about childbirth. They were afraid of forthcoming pain, the risk of infection and the possibility of their own death, or that of their baby. Their apprehensions may also have been compounded with concerns about the practicalities and costs of bringing up a new child.

Dr Robert Gooch (1784–1830), an eminent London general practitioner and obstetrician, made the first detailed medical diagnosis of 'puerperal insanity' in 1819. There was an increasing interest in the condition from the medical profession during the ensuing decades. In the nineteenth century, Puerperal Insanity was also known as 'insanity of childbirth' and sometimes as 'lactational insanity' (when there was a slightly later onset if problems arose around breast feeding). This was a serious and debilitating mental disorder that could affect normal, peaceful and caring women from all levels of society and it could also exacerbate the health of women who already had a predisposition to mental illness. It was often characterised by a disastrously rapid onset of symptoms triggered by childbirth, or within six weeks of it. In its extreme form some deaths were attributed to puerperal insanity, with several affected mothers struggling with urges to kill themselves, their husbands, or their newborn infants. Some mothers did commit infanticide.

Nevertheless, puerperal insanity was generally considered to be a temporary and entirely curable illness with a good prognosis. Most women made a complete recovery within a few months. Puerperal insanity could appear after the birth of any child in a family, not necessarily the first-born, and could recur in subsequent deliveries. The onset was considered more likely if there had been complications in the confinement such as the birth of a stillborn child, a prolonged or difficult labour, the unexpected occurrence of twins, or the need for surgical intervention in the labour such as the use of forceps.

The medical profession divided puerperal insanity into two categories: puerperal melancholia, a depressive disorder not considered particularly unusual and which is now known as 'post-natal depression'; and puerperal mania which was a far more devastating psychological disorder, today known as 'puerperal psychosis', distinguished by over-excitement, risky, erratic, dangerous and disturbingly deviant behaviour. Symptoms could include self-neglect, restlessness, sexual disinhibition and violence.

John Haslam, as apothecary to the Bethlehem Hospital in London, recorded eighty cases of puerperal insanity admitted there between 1784 and 1794. Women with puerperal mania were far more likely to be admitted to an asylum than those suffering puerperal melancholia, who could usually be managed at home unless their level of depression was severe.

For those with puerperal mania, their psychoses could manifest in many different ways. Textbooks of psychological medicine from the mid-nineteenth century record that women suffering from puerperal madness could demonstrate:

> *a total negligence of, and often very strong aversion to her child and husband ... explosions of anger occur, with vociferations and violent gesticulations and, although the patient may have been remarkable previously for her correct, modest demeanour, and attention to her religious duties, most awful oaths and imprecations are now uttered, and language used which astonishes her friends. ... she might show a great degree of excitement ... with a lively propensity to every kind of mischief.*

At the beginning of the nineteenth century obstetricians felt that they, rather than alienists, were the authorities on puerperal insanity. However, as the century progressed with an increase in the number of asylums and the recognition of the medical profession of psychiatry, puerperal insanity fell under the remit of alienists. In 1872, Sir James Young Simpson (1811–70), the obstetrician who pioneered the use of chloroform as an anaesthetic in childbirth, estimated that ten per cent of all female lunatic asylum admissions were attributed to puerperal insanity.

Case study: Eliza Straffen

Eliza Straffen, a 41-year-old vicar's wife from Coventry, was admitted to the private asylum at Ticehurst, Sussex in April 1868 with suicidal mania caused by childbirth and an inability to suckle her child. Her admission notes recorded that she was 'screaming, struggling, biting, and trying to throw herself and her attendants down to the ground'. She spat in attendants' faces and expressed violent delusions of being burnt and being blind. Eliza attempted suicide by putting her head out of windows and letting the sash fall on to it. She tied a handkerchief around her neck in an attempt to strangle herself. She also tried to swallow it and crammed a lot of paper in her mouth in order to choke herself. Eliza threw her attendant to the ground and tried to strangle her and it took three or four attendants to restrain her.

Eliza was placed in a warm bath for thirty minutes with cold compresses applied to her head, and was given liquid opium every hour. After two doses she became quieter and remained on regular oral morphine for the next six weeks before being weaned off it. She was discharged 'recovered' after four months in Ticehurst.

Case Study: Catherine Jeffers

Catherine Jeffers, a 21-year-old married housewife from Manchester, became very violent one month after giving birth to her first child in April 1872. She was admitted to an asylum with puerperal mania on 17 May 1872. Her asylum admission notes record that she was very violent, rather excited and restless, spat at, bit and kicked, everybody who went near her. Catherine refused to take her food and believed that she was in Heaven and everyone around her were angels. She was unable to understand where she was, or why she was there.

Within a week she had calmed down, was much quieter, had rested well and was described as 'sensible'. On 27 June 1872 the asylum doctor recorded 'a most wonderful improvement'. As her husband intended to take her to the seaside to convalesce, she was discharged 'recovered'.

Case study: Esther Hooper

Esther Hooper was a 36-year-old housekeeper from Bolton, Lancashire who threatened to destroy herself and her child six weeks after giving birth. Her husband described her as 'completely changed'. On admission to an asylum on 30 November 1872, the medical case notes record that she was rather incoherent in speech and became excited when she was spoken to. She was considered both suicidal and dangerous. A diagnosis of puerperal mania was made and it was noted that she had a hereditary predisposition to insanity.

In the first few weeks of her admission, Esther's sister, Nancy Hardman, informed the medical officer that Esther had always been of a nervous disposition. 'Since her confinement her husband had been drinking hard and that her home was anything but comfortable and she did not get enough support in her weak state.'

Esther was reluctant to return home despite her rapid progress once under the comfortable care of the asylum. She worked happily in the sewing room, but wished to remain in the asylum until the medical staff considered her to be strong. Esther was discharged 'recovered' on 25 January 1873 having gained weight and bodily health.

She appears on the 1881 census at 156, Church Street, Bolton, with her 8-year-old daughter, Grace; they were living with her unmarried elder sister Nancy, who was an organist and teacher of music.

Case study: Sarah Fullard

Sarah Fullard was a 20-year-old married weaver admitted to Parkside Asylum on 22 June 1872. She appeared to be 'a young woman with an exceedingly morose expression of countenance, constipated and in a very bad temper.' She was suffering from violent excitement, could not control herself and made an attempt to knock the doctor's hat off in the waiting room. The day after admission she struck another patient with a chamber pot and was moved out of the dormitory into a single room. She was diagnosed with puerperal mania.

A month later there was little or no improvement and she remained sullen and obstinate. By September there was only little progress – she remained morose and would not speak for several days at a time. By the middle of November however, she began to improve and was anxious to return home to care for her children. She was discharged on trial on 21 November 1872 and by 22 December was considered 'recovered'.

Case Study: Thomasine Entwistle

On 5 November 1873, Thomasine Entwistle, a 37-year-old married housewife from Manchester was admitted to an asylum ten days after giving birth. She talked incoherently, continually undressed herself and refused to stay in bed. When spoken to she replied in a very sulky manner and regularly used bad language. On admission she was noted as being physically weak due to her recent confinement. She was diagnosed with puerperal mania but made a speedy recovery and was discharged deemed recovered after twenty-three days.

Treatment

Obstetricians were generally opposed to asylum treatment, preferring private seclusion and good nursing care unless the patient was dangerous, suicidal or unmanageable, or if her illness became prolonged. Alienists agreed that milder cases did not require asylum treatment.

Therapy involved removing the mother from her home and family and placing her in a safe, tranquil and supporting environment in an asylum. Mothers were separated from their babies and were encouraged to rest while being provided with a good, nourishing diet. Forced feeding with a stomach pump was sometimes used for women who refused to eat, particularly in the latter decades of the century. Suicidal cases were watched carefully. In cases of extreme restlessness or violence, sedation was used. Medical treatments evolved as the century progressed. Constipation tended to be an issue with women who had recently given birth due to dehydration, so laxatives or 'purgatives' were administered freely.

While their mothers were detained in the asylum, many of the newborn infants were looked after by family members. Wealthy families would engage a private nurse while in poorer families, the infant could be boarded out and cared for by other women under the Poor Law system. There was no facility for keeping babies in asylums and those born there were removed.

Case studies: Janet Smith and Eliza Paterson

Janet Smith, a 23-year-old married woman from the city of Edinburgh was admitted to the Royal Edinburgh Asylum in April 1853 with puerperal mania. She had become insane ten days after a prolonged labour, which had culminated in a traumatic forceps delivery of a live child – her first delivery. Janet became restless, wild, destructive, and uncontrollable and was initially treated with an anodyne of morphine and hyoscine. Because of her hot-headedness her scalp was shaved and blisters were applied to the nape of her neck (see Chapter 19 *Treatments*). Her breasts, which had become full, were rubbed with Oil of Camphor.

Eliza Paterson, a 25-year-old married woman, was admitted to the Royal Edinburgh Asylum in July 1855 suffering from puerperal melancholia after the birth of her second child. She had attempted suicide by self-strangulation with a shawl tied tightly around her neck on the day prior to admission. She was treated with 'tonics and laxatives', her hair was cut closely to her scalp and her head blistered, and she was enveloped in wet sheets with a note that she was to be watched closely.

Infanticide
The rate of infanticide in cases of puerperal insanity was quite low. Throughout the nineteenth century a number of unmarried mothers, particularly young servant girls, concealed their pregnancies and killed their newborn infants at, or shortly after, birth and hid the bodies. This was sometimes regarded as a solution to the social stigma of having an illegitimate child, and all the economic burdens this involved. Prior to the 1803 *Offences Against the Person Act*, infanticide was a capital offence; the mother was presumed guilty of murder and would be sentenced to death by judicial hanging unless she could prove that the child had been stillborn. By the 1803 Act, a mother who killed her child would be charged with murder, but was presumed innocent until proven otherwise. The Act took into account the possibility of stillbirth, or death of the neonate by natural causes, and allowed juries to return a verdict of 'concealment of birth', which carried a maximum penalty of two years imprisonment. Most cases of infanticide thereafter were acquitted or found guilty of the lesser offence of concealment. Puerperal insanity began to be used with increasing frequency as a defence plea in cases of infanticide or concealment.

Both forms of puerperal insanity – melancholia and mania – could lead to infanticide. Melancholia could lead to apathy and neglect, whereas mania could cause unexpected, catastrophic, and violent mood changes with sudden, unpredictable, explosive behaviour.

Case study: Hannah Sullivan

Hannah Sullivan was a 17-year-old Catholic domestic servant from County Cork, Ireland, when, in December 1895, she was indicted at the Munster Winter Assizes, Cork, for the wilful murder of her illegitimate, male child. According to her case records, she killed the baby 'by cutting off its head in a loft in her master's premises at Tralee.' Hannah claimed that she did not realise that she was giving birth and the baby's head got stuck in the toilet seat. The jury found that Hannah had committed the act while insane. She was ordered to be detained at Her Majesty's pleasure at Dundrum Criminal Lunatic Asylum. Hannah was discharged to her mother one year later with no residual signs of insanity.

Chapter 17

Suicide

Suicidal patients were one of the most important and fragile groups admitted to lunatic asylums. Asylums had a duty of care to protect these vulnerable people by providing them with a place of safe custody and ensuring they had full physical and mental support. Suicidal patients often acted irrationally and on impulse, sometimes fuelled by alcohol or other stimulants. Admitting them to an asylum and allowing them a 'cool-down' period provided them not only with a place of safety where they could reflect on their fears and their future, but also an opportunity to be psychiatrically assessed and counselled by the only available professionals in the nineteenth century – the asylum doctors. After discussion and reflection, most patients chose life rather than death.

When someone threatened, or more seriously attempted suicide, the immediate action to be taken by families, medical practitioners, police, poor law officials or the clergy was clear – the only sensible option was to preserve life by committal of the afflicted person to a place of safety – an asylum. During the course of the nineteenth century between one-quarter and one-third of all patients admitted to a lunatic asylum in the British Isles were described as 'suicidal' on their admission papers. Being suicidal was certainly seen as a compulsory reason for admission to an asylum. One eminent English alienist, Sir George Henry Savage (1842–1921), chief medical officer of Bethlehem Royal Hospital, London, believed that this figure was a gross exaggeration, and that the true rate of what he termed 'actively suicidal' patients – being those 'who have made serious attempts on their lives, and likely to repeat them' – was actually no more than five per cent.

In a study of patients admitted to the Roxburgh District Lunatic Asylum in the last quarter of the nineteenth century, it was shown that males opted for more violent means to commit suicide such as hanging themselves, or cutting their throats or wrists, as these methods had a more likely chance of success. Females tended to prefer self-poisoning or impulsive, attention-seeking behaviours such as jumping into a fire or running in front of a moving vehicle often as a 'cry for help' rather than a determined desire to kill themselves.

This category of patient was placed on 'suicide watch' on their admission to an asylum where they would be closely observed by their attendants. This close watch was only relaxed once the authorities thought the risk of suicide had diminished. Belts, braces, neckties, and bootlaces were removed so that these could not be used for self-strangulation. Meals could only be eaten with a blunt spoon as knives and forks were considered dangerous. Men were not allowed to use razors to shave, and the majority of photographs of male patients show them with ever lengthening beards. Actively suicidal patients were put in 'strong clothes' and provided with 'strong sheets' on their beds, which could not be torn into strips. Those considered at highest risk of suicide were sometimes placed in straightjackets. In certain cases sedating medication was prescribed.

Asylums were constructed to maximise the safety of their patients, which was particularly important for those deemed to be suicidal. From the mid-nineteenth century asylums were built to designs that maximised patient safety, security and comfort. The asylum in Glasgow was built following a radial design that allowed attendants to observe patients at all times. Staircases and windows were also designed with the suicidal patient in mind, so that they could not jump over handrails, smash window glass, or hang themselves on window cords. The need to supervise a large number of suicidal patients in a confined space meant it was important that any possible methods of potential suicide should be minimised to reduce the risk to patient life. As a result, medical superintendents and architects were careful in their choice of design of a new asylum. They were also mindful that however suicide-proof a building appeared to be, without the constant vigilance of asylum attendants, the most determined of patients could succeed in ending their own lives. Not only was this an undesirable outcome for the patient, it was also not good for asylum staff who were accountable to the Lunacy Commissioners for their care of the insane. Asylum handbooks written for the guidance of attendants stressed the importance of ensuring the safety of all patients, but particularly those deemed to be suicidal. Attendants could be charged with negligence if they failed to follow the guidelines. The telltale clock requiring attendants to 'clock-in' at various intervals, and other similar devices ensured that they remained vigilant during night shifts. Some asylums had inspection plates on the doors of single rooms so that patients could be observed discreetly.

Asylums saw the prevention of suicide as one of their prime objectives. However, many patients attempted, or successfully managed, to commit suicide whilst in-patients in asylums.

Case studies: suicides

Sarah Ann Bennet was 33 years old and an unmarried, silk millworker when she was admitted to the Cheshire Asylum on 24 April 1894. On examination it was noted that she had attempted to strangle herself. She was described as violent, quarrelsome, noisy and uncontrollable, sometimes requiring seclusion or 'to be held'. However, on 23 November 1895, Sarah Ann tied a garter tightly around her neck and was found 'black in her face' but was cut down by an attendant. She survived that attempt on her life, but attempted the same method on two subsequent occasions both of which were prevented thanks to the vigilance of the asylum attendants.

Mary Phillips, a 59-year-old farmer's wife, had attempted suicide three times before being admitted to Carmarthen Lunatic Asylum in March 1870 with severe depression – twice with a knife and once with a rope. She was being closely watched on her ward but, on 18 May 1870, she managed to go to a part of the asylum where she should not have been and strangled herself with copper wire round her neck attached to a lavatory seat. At the coroner's inquest the attendants were found 'much to blame' for her death.

Robert Ruthven, a 25-year-old married woodman from Selkirk, was admitted to Roxburgh District Asylum in February 1895 suffering from acute melancholia. Initially, he was placed in seclusion in a strong room and prescribed chloral hydrate and potassium bromide. Robert continued to have delusions that people accused him of having sex with cows and chasing sheep. Whilst out on a working party in the grounds of the asylum in November 1895, Robert managed to poison himself by ingesting a huge quantity of nails and yew leaves. The cause of death on his death certificate is rather explicit – 'Failure of the action of the heart, due to the presence in his stomach of 9 ¾ ounces of metal nails and other pieces of metal, and to the poisonous effects of a quantity of yew leaves swallowed with suicidal intent.' The subsequent Record of Corrected Entries confirms that death was caused by 'irritant poison (suicidal)'.

Mark O'Connor, a 27-year-old single man, was admitted to Cork Asylum in April 1896 as a dangerous lunatic suffering from acute melancholia. He had attempted suicide twice before admission – once by strangulation, and once by cutting his throat. He was placed on 'suicide watch' in the observation ward. On 24 May 1896, when the two attendants supervising thirteen suicidal patients were busy making beds, he slipped out of the dormitory. Some minutes later he was found suspended by a necktie from one of the downpipes in the toilet block.

On Sunday 11 December 1898, a group of patients were being marched back to their quarters at the Connacht District Asylum at Ballinasloe, County Galway, after attending Mass accompanied by several keepers. One of them, Michael Mannian of Kiltormer, made a sudden dash from the ranks, ran at full speed for the River Suck at the back of the asylum 200yds away and plunged into the water head first. After removing his boots, one of the keepers dived in after Mannian but could not reach him. The water was very deep at that particular spot and the body was recovered some hours later.

There were also a number of patients who were admitted to asylums in a suicidal state and who were subsequently discharged deemed 'recovered', and who went on to commit successful suicides within a few months after their discharge.

Case study: Andrew Shiels
Andrew Shiels was a 56-year-old millworker in 1886. Sadly, two of his daughters, Helen Mary and Mariann, had died in infancy, and his youngest daughter, Martha, died in May 1877 at the age of 11 from typhoid fever. When Andrew's wife died in 1884 he became severely depressed. He felt life was not worth living and so, on 25 May 1886, Andrew took an overdose of laudanum expecting to opt out of life. He woke up, despondent to be alive, and tried to cut his throat. Again this was unsuccessful – he did not cut deep enough. Andrew was admitted to the Roxburgh District Asylum. By 30 June 1886 he appeared 'cheerful and

sensible' and was discharged. Four months later he successfully committed suicide by stabbing himself in the neck in his daughter's house on a night that he knew the family were out. He had placed a pail between his knees to catch the blood to prevent making a mess on her floor.

In nineteenth century England and Wales suicide was illegal. Those who tried and failed could be charged with attempted self-murder, and anyone who assisted or abetted them could also be charged as accessories to their crime. By the 1870s, an average of over 800 people a year were being arrested in England and Wales for attempted suicide, rising to over a thousand a year in the 1890s. However, only a small percentage of the thousands arrested were actually committed for trial. In England and Wales suicide was condemned a mortal sin in the eyes of the Church and the law. Those who succeeded were guilty of a crime known as *felo de se* – a felon of oneself. The implication of this was that, prior to 1823, people guilty of *felo de se* could not receive a Christian burial in consecrated ground. The Church's view was that they had violated the Church's belief that life was a God-given gift and not for man to take away. The burial restrictions were relaxed by the 1823 *Burial of Suicide Act* and the 1882 *Interments (felo de se) Act*.

In Ireland, suicide was also an indictable crime and police constables were advised that persons who attempted suicide were to be arrested and charged with an offence. In Scotland, under Scots Law, suicide itself was not an offence but a person attempting suicide could be charged with a 'breach of the peace' and anyone assisting a suicide could be charged with murder or culpable homicide.

Case studies
In December 1893 a 33-year-old mother of six appeared in court in Birmingham charged with attempting to commit suicide. The previous month she had obtained a revolver and several cartridges and, while standing in front of a looking glass, had fired the gun into her mouth. The bullet passed through the back of her throat and lodged itself in her head but did not kill her. She was admitted to hospital and following her discharge was tried in court under criminal law despite not having recovered and looking extremely unwell. The judge believed she had suffered enough and allowed her home to the care of her relatives. Shortly

afterwards she was admitted to Birmingham City Asylum where she died on 17 December 1902 of General Paralysis of the Insane.

On Saturday 14 November 1874, Louisa Hat or Fraser, a 30-year-old widow, was brought before Sheriff Frederick Hallard at the City Police Court in Edinburgh charged with attempting to commit suicide by jumping into a mill lade early the previous morning. At the request of the public officer of health, who said she was afflicted with insanity although not a dangerous lunatic, the hearing was postponed to the following Monday and she was transferred to Morningside Asylum suffering from mental depression. There, on Sunday 15 November, she tore a bed-sheet into strips and strangled herself with one of them.

As the nineteenth century progressed, the view that suicide was a moral offence changed. It became accepted that people who attempted suicide were sick. Suicide was finally decriminalised in England and Wales in 1961 by the *Suicide Act – An Act to amend the law of England and Wales relating to suicide, and for the purposes connected therewith*. The same law was enacted verbatim in *Criminal Justice (Northern Ireland) Act* of 1966 for Northern Ireland. The Act did not apply to Scotland, as suicide was never an offence under Scots law.

Chapter 18

Diagnoses and Causes

In the last quarter of the nineteenth century alienists in Britain and Ireland developed a classification agreed by the Medico-Psychological Association (MPA) to define, record and analyse the diagnoses and causes of insanity of patients admitted to asylums. Dr David Skae (1814–73), medical superintendent of the Royal Edinburgh Asylum from 1846–73, had previously developed a more complicated system of categorising diagnoses, published in 1863. In some institutions, such as the Royal Edinburgh, patients were given two diagnoses – one from the MPA classification and one from Dr Skae's.

Diagnoses
Diagnoses as defined by the Medico-Psychological Association were:

- Mania
- Melancholia
- General Paralysis of the Insane
- Epileptic Mania
- Congenital defect with epilepsy
- Congenital defect without epilepsy
- Dementia

Skae's classification was more specific and was not agreed by all alienists with some of the diagnoses being controversial. His diagnoses were:

- Congenital Insanity
- Epileptic Insanity
- Insanity of Adolescence
- Climateric (Menopausal) Insanity
- Senile Insanity

- Insanity of Pregnancy
- Puerperal Insanity
- Insanity of Lactation
- Hysterical Insanity
- Uterine Insanity
- Insanity of Masturbation
- General Paralysis
- Insanity of Brain Disease
- Traumatic Insanity
- Syphilitic Insanity
- Anaemic Insanity
- Phthisical Insanity
- Insanity of Alcohol
- Post-febrile Insanity
- Idiopathic Insanity
- Insanity of Unknown Cause.

The commonest diagnoses of those admitted to asylums using the traditional MPA classification were mania and melancholia (either acute or chronic), followed by general paralysis and dementia.

Mania

Mania was a catastrophic and alarming form of acute mental illness. It was a form of abrupt insanity characterised by 'mental exaltation and bodily excitement'. It usually had a very quick and totally unpredictable onset. In its acute form, symptoms could manifest as a disastrous loss of self-control, restlessness, loquacity, incoherent speech, foolish and irrational misconduct, unstable mood, a complete inability to sleep, an excitable temper, and the voicing of delusions and hallucinations. Patients could demonstrate 'a rapid flow of ideas, with inability to fix their attention … exhibiting unmeaning happiness, passing into uproarious hilarity'. There was display of pressure of thought, pressure of ideas and an inability to focus. Sufferers would speak rapidly and irrationally with varying and unconnected ideas. Acute mania could lead to rapid exhaustion.

The chronic form of mania manifested itself in a condition of mental exaltation for a prolonged period of time in which patients presented exacerbations of restlessness, excitability and destructive behaviours.

Case study: Jane Winstanley

Jane Winstanley, a 25-year-old grocer's wife, was admitted to Parkside Asylum, Cheshire, on 16 June 1886 with a three-day history of extreme excitement. The admission notes record 'eyes rolling and staring, turning head rapidly from side to side, throwing herself on the ground needlessly unless held, running about with indifference, fights and struggles violently when held, very noisy, shouting and muttering inarticulate sounds, pays no heed to anything said to her'. She required force-feeding with a stomach pump. One week later, Jane was expressing delusions of having a menagerie of animals passing over her when in bed, and that she was going to have her eyes put out. Jane remained in the asylum for six months.

Case study: John Oldfield

John Oldfield was admitted to an asylum in September 1896 suffering from acute mania. He was a police sergeant who had been in the force for over twenty-five years. He was considered dangerous because he had threatened to shoot people. The medical superintendent recorded that he had known John for some time and 'always considered him to be eccentric'. His mania was so acute that it took six attendants to take him to the ward.

Once calm, John was able to explain that sunstroke followed by rheumatic fever had weakened him, thus preventing him from executing his official duties to full effect. He had been involved in an unpleasant rape case during which he was bullied by a senior police officer. This culminated in a request for him to report to headquarters where he was informed he had to stand trial in front of a Police Committee. This news upset him greatly causing a mental breakdown and his admission.

John's mental health began to improve and he became calmer and less worried about his situation. He was 'relieved' from the asylum, deemed 'recovered', in November 1896.

Melancholia

Melancholia was defined as 'the expression of a feeling of misery for which no sufficient justification exists'. This was a manifestation of clinical depression. Patients often presented with a number of symptoms predominated by low mood. They would present with a bowed head and a flattened facial expression, showing no emotion. This would be accompanied by general inertia or lethargy. Patients may have exhibited a loss of appetite, been in low spirits and demonstrated a general uneasiness and signs of self-neglect. The individual's refusal to eat could lead to constipation. The depressed mood could lead to thoughts of death and suicide. Acute melancholia could be a reaction to life events such as the death of a child or a spouse. Melancholia was considered to be a condition very liable to relapse. Cases of melancholia were classified as either acute or chronic according to their duration; any case that culminated within a few weeks would be labelled acute melancholia.

Case study: William Fleming

William Fleming was a 37-year-old married weaver working in Hawick in the Scottish Borders. Previously a 'constant and industrious worker', William shunned away from his employment in March of 1890. During the next month he became increasingly gloomy, despondent, and reclusive. He said he was tired of life and wished he were dead. A kitchen knife was found under his pillow precipitating his admission to Roxburgh District Asylum. On admission he was noted to be 'considerably depressed', with the appearance of 'a thin pale melancholic man'. William was discharged back to his family as 'recovered' after four months in the asylum.

Case study: Jabez Taylor

Jabez Ramsden Taylor was admitted as a private patient to an asylum on 24 April 1891 as a result of over-study. Jabez was a 21-year-old medical student at Edinburgh University and was described as a 'thin delicate looking lad with hollow cheeks'. Pampered by an indulgent mother, Jabez was timid and hesitating and lacked self-confidence. He was sent to Edinburgh to study medicine at the age of 16. Being removed from all his friends, Jabez struggled to cope on his own. His memory deteriorated and he had difficulty collecting his thoughts, which resulted in melancholia. After a year in the asylum, Jabez was relieved in May 1892.

Dementia

A diagnosis of 'dementia' in nineteenth century Britain was very different to its definition today. Dementia referred to an acquired mental failing of the brain due to disease or decay. Many people who were diagnosed with dementia in the nineteenth century would have been diagnosed with affective disorders such as schizophrenia or bipolar disease in the following centuries. Some could be suffering from the later stages of General Paralysis of the Insane. Dementia was classified as: primary (acute), secondary (following attacks of acute or chronic mania or melancholia), or senile (age related). Primary dementia was insidious in onset and typically the patient would gradually acquire a few harmless delusions; although tractable and docile, they would be useless in the grade of society to which they belonged. Senile dementia was seen as simply an exaggeration of the decay of the system from advancing years – with the major symptom being a loss of short-term memory, while retaining memories of what happened long ago. These patients tended to demonstrate a loss of insight to time or place.

Case study: Albert Sidebottom
Albert Sidebottom was a 40-year-old former railway clerk who was admitted to Parkside on 17 May 1871 having previously been in the asylums of Chester and Cheadle. He had delusions regarding property, money, horses and marriage and had ordered a great many items that he did not need. He was diagnosed with dementia, and the pre-disposing cause of sunstroke three years earlier was given as a reason for his mental state. He was a tall, thin man with a delicate appearance and was put on cod liver oil on admission. His physical condition weakened and he was given a dose of porter and milk in the evenings to help sustain him. Albert died on 15 February 1873 from 'softening of the brain'.

Case study: Mary Archer
Mary Archer, a 62-year-old widow from Ashton-under-Lyne, was admitted to an asylum on 5 October 1872 with a diagnosis of senile dementia. On admission she appeared restless, nervous, weak and physically exhausted. Mary was constantly muttering to herself and seemed to be saying 'I must dance out my salvation'. She was, literally, tearing her hair out, pulling at her clothes, and stripping herself naked. Because of her restlessness and weak state, Mary was prescribed chloral hydrate as a sedative and was ordered to have beef tea and two ounces of wine daily to build her up. Although the chloral calmed her down, there was little change in her general mental state after a month in the asylum, and she started to show signs of erysipelas on her face – a bacterial skin infection. At that time, the cause of erysipelas was not known and was

thought to be due to poor sanitation. As part of her treatment, her red, hot, swollen face was covered with cotton wadding and she was prescribed one teaspoon of whisky every three hours. Mary gradually 'sank' and died on 8 November 1872.

General Paralysis of the Insane, Epilepsy, and Congenital Insanity (Imbeciles and Idiots) are addressed in separate chapters.

Causes

The Medical Psychological Association divided the causes into 'predisposing', which were mainly physical; and 'exciting', which they termed 'moral'. Patients could have both predisposing and exciting causes for their illness, and more than one of each. Moral causes of insanity greatly exceeded physical ones.

The predisposing (physical) causes included:

- A hereditary predisposition
- Consanguineous parents (cousin marriages)
- A great difference in age between parents
- Congenital defects
- Birth trauma
- Head injury
- Brain disease
- Epilepsy
- Puberty
- Pregnancy, childbirth and lactation
- The climacteric (menopause)
- Menstrual disorders
- Old age
- Fever and febrile illnesses (such as acute urinary tract infection, measles, typhoid or tuberculosis/consumption)
- Chronic physical ill-health (including gout, rheumatism, heart disease, asthma, phthisis and syphilis)
- Privation and starvation
- Intense heat (sunstroke)
- Intense cold (hypothermia)
- Poisoning (including lead and mercury)

The moral causes included:

- Intemperance of alcohol, tobacco, opium or other substances
- Religious anxiety, excitement and 'spiritualism'
- Intense study
- Overwork
- Disappointment in love (including love thwarted and jealousy)
- Family affections
- Domestic troubles (including drunkenness of a family member, ill-treatment, or desertion)
- Domestic grief (illness or death of a relative or friend)
- Sexual vice, including masturbation
- Disappointed ambition
- Adverse circumstances (including business anxieties and pecuniary difficulties)
- Political excitement and war
- Fear and fright ('nervous shock')
- Sudden change from a life of idleness
- Imprisonment or solitary confinement

The Famine of 1845–49 in Ireland was also a trigger to many cases of mental illness. Following this period, some of the Irish asylum superintendents believed tea to be an exciting cause, particularly if it had been left 'stewing' at length.

Chapter 19

Treatments

Mechanical restraint

Restraint was one of the most widely used methods to deal with insanity until, and during, the eighteenth century, particularly for violent patients. The restraint of troublesome lunatics was not intended as a treatment, but rather as a method to punish, control and discipline them and to confine them in a place where they could not harm others. The patients were treated no better than dangerous, wild beasts – and were caged or restrained by a variety of means including manacles, fetters, handcuffs, leather straps, straight-jackets, leg irons and iron collars placed around the neck. Many lunatics were chained to a wall or to an iron bedstead at night. They were kept in dark rooms or cells so that they were 'not affected by the stimulus of light'. Consideration was given to their carers to minimise the burden and anxiety of dealing with unruly lunatics.

Straight waistcoats (also known as straight-jackets) were used to immobilise patients. They were most frequently made of strong canvas material; the patient's arms were placed into long sleeves that were tied tightly to their trunk. A similar method applied to those who were 'disposed to tear clothes or strike others was the application of leather mitts on the hands, attached to a leather belt around the waist.' Leather mitts were also used to prevent patients making themselves vomit by placing their fingers down their throats. Some maternity patients were made to wear two layers of stockings and had their legs bandaged together to stop them kicking out.

Mechanical restraint was still being used in the early nineteenth century when it was gradually replaced by moral treatment. Straight-jackets were used alongside moral therapy and continued in use during the twentieth century.

Seclusion

In the pre-asylum era, lunatics were often confined and hidden in outhouses, attics or cellars to be 'out of sight and out of mind'. Later, seclusion was used as part of the moral therapy within the asylum to place patients guilty of violent and unmanageable behaviours in temporary isolation, usually in a solitary cell. This was aimed to calm them down, prevent them abusing staff and other patients, and also deter them from reoffending. There was a belief that removing a patient from the environment that had caused their madness would be beneficial. It provided tranquillity in a quiet space rather than being exposed to a crowd of other patients. Most asylums had padded cells or rooms into which suicidal patients could be placed for their own safety, where the chances of harming themselves by punching or head-butting the walls were minimalised. Padded cells were particularly effective for epileptic patients or for those experiencing violent maniacal episodes; such cells were introduced to the basement wards of London's Bethlehem Hospital in 1844 and were viewed as more punitive than therapeutic. At other times, however, allowing patients to walk about alone in one of the airing courts was also used as a therapeutic method of seclusion.

Case study: Elizabeth Lingard

Elizabeth Lingard, a 28-year-old single woman, was admitted to Parkside Asylum on 16 August 1882 with a diagnosis of epileptic insanity, having been in a workhouse for the previous eight years. She was described as having a 'bad character' and her case notes show that she spent many repeated episodes secluded in the padded room and was regularly restrained by up to six nurses when 'furiously excited'. Her manic behaviour coincided with epileptic seizures. She died on 24 September 1885 from epileptiform convulsions.

Heroic – balancing the humours

The Greek physician Hippocrates of Kos (circa 460–357 BC), argued that every human body was composed of, and was controlled by, a system of four basic 'vital spirits' or 'humours' that interacted with one another – blood (making the body warm and moist); phlegm (making the body cold and wet); black bile (making the body cold and dry); and, yellow bile (making the body hot and dry). His theory was that the relative balance of these humours influenced the physical and emotional wellbeing of an individual. Where there was an imbalance of too much blood, it produced a florid complexion and made one 'sanguine' and hot tempered; too much phlegm rendered one pale and phlegmatic or apathetic; too much yellow bile made one bilious or choleric, bringing on aggression; and an excess of black bile gave one a dark complexion with melancholia (in Greek 'black bile' is μέλαινα χολή, *melaina chole*).

Excesses of blood or yellow bile would lead to mania, whereas an excess of black bile, being cold and dry, resulted in lowness and depression. This theory still held in the sixteenth century when it was thought the harmful humours had an effect on the brain.

Where there was an excess of any of these four humours the balance needed to be restored by drawing out the excessive one. Good health could only be achieved by keeping the humours in equilibrium. These theories went out of favour in the early nineteenth century when moral treatment and a greater understanding of medicine became the recognised approach to treating the insane.

Bleeding

Bleeding or blood-letting, which was effected either by the sucking out of blood by leeches, or by the lancing of veins (phlebotomy or venesection), was used to balance the humours if it appeared that there was an excess of blood. Leeches were placed on the forehead, behind the ears, or in the nostrils, to relieve melancholic congestion of the brain. They were placed around the genitalia and inner thighs to treat puerperal mania. Lancing was used when there were symptoms of brain inflammation or congestion leading to mania.

Blistering

This technique of capillary bleeding was also known as 'cupping'. Blistering was achieved by applying heated cups to the body to raise blisters which were applied in order to 'draw out the noxious humours' – mainly yellow phlegm – as part of the treatment for puerperal insanity. The resultant blisters were scratched with specialised surgical instruments to release the noxious effluents. Mustard poultices to the legs and thighs with warm baths were being used the 1860s. They could also be applied to the nape of the neck. 'Cataplasms' were poultices, sometimes warmed and medicated, which were applied over the skin.

Emetics and Purgatives

The humoural doctrine linked the gastrointestinal tract, where the humours were replenished by digestion and expelled when exhausted, with some forms of insanity. Emetics were medicines or potions, often herbal remedies, given to a patient to induce vomiting to 'empty the stomach of the accumulation of bodily toxins'. Besides the humoural theory, many asylum patients were constipated as a result of poor diet or from the side effects of medication, particularly opiates. Purgatives, as herbal remedies, roots, salts or oils were used as laxatives to clear out the bowels. Castor oil and Epsom salts were frequently used. There are many natural laxatives including senna, rhubarb, and prunes. An 1851 textbook on Obstetrics advised purging of the bowel in cases of puerperal insanity.

> *Many cases have occurred where the disease has almost instantaneously given way to the thorough evacuation of the* [bowel]. *In such, the matters expelled have been in excessive quantity, most unhealthy and offensive, and were evidently the exciting cases of the derangement.*

Bowels could also be evacuated by the use of suppositories or enemas.

Shaving the head

Shaving the head was periodically used to treat hot-headed individuals with a view 'to lessen the heat'. Cataplasms were then applied to the shaved scalp to stimulate the brain for additional therapeutic benefit. These were made from a variety of different substances depending on the preferred method of the prescribing physician. Lavender was used for its calming effects.

Bathing (hydrotherapy)

Forced immersions by ducking the patient's head in a tub of cold water until they nearly drowned and 'baths of surprise' were used early in the nineteenth century to stimulate fear to bring patients 'back to reality'. In the latter form of coercion, the patient was made to walk, either in the dark or blindfolded, along a passage that had a bath of icy cold water under a trap-door into which they fell without warning.

The therapeutic use of water involved various forms of baths, showers, douches, and footbaths at varying temperatures, used to soothe, subdue or invigorate patients as well as cleanse them. Prolonged warm or hot baths, for thirty minutes to an hour, were most frequently used for cases of mania, nervous irritability and insomnia. Cold baths were rarely used, but applications to the head from cold wet towels, jugs of cold water poured over the head or ice packs, whilst the body or just the feet were placed in warm water, were thought to be advantageous by cooling the brain.

Tepid baths into which crude mustard was dissolved were occasionally used in some asylums and found to be effective in cases of severe mania. Mustard baths were believed to lower body temperature and decrease blood circulation and Samuel Newington (1739–1811), the founder of Ticehurst Asylum in Sussex, was a firm promoter of their use. The patient was placed in the bath for thirty minutes and was usually 'perfectly red upon being taken out'. They could, however, cause skin irritation, particularly to the genitals.

Prolonged cold showers were also used until, in April 1856, Daniel Dolley, a patient in the Surrey County Lunatic Asylum, died after spending twenty-eight minutes in a cold shower; the Commissioners in Lunacy subsequently issued instructions restricting their use to a maximum of three minutes.

Dietary remedies

A change of diet was often used to treat maniacal insanity. Lunatics could be put on a 'diluting' or 'cooling' diet of green vegetables, barley water and milk. 'Sanguine' patients, thought to have an excess of the humour of blood, were banned from wine and red meat. Meat was considered 'to inflame the passions'. John Conolly noted in 1856 that, prior to moral therapy, many asylum patients suffered from *scorbutus* – this was an alternative name for scurvy caused by vitamin C deficiency.

Weak patients could be prescribed milk, wine, raw eggs or beef tea to 'beef them up'. Many pauper patients were poorly nourished and a wholesome nutritious diet was seen as part of their treatment. Underweight patients were often prescribed 'extras' above the normal asylum rations. Thomas Clouston, medical superintendent of the Royal Edinburgh Asylum, noted that all acute mental diseases 'tend to thinness of body' and he preached a 'gospel of fatness'. Liquid custards made of eggs and milk were given twice daily to underweight patients.

Many paupers had rotten or missing teeth that caused difficulties with biting or chewing their food so they were given either a soft diet or minced food. Dental decay could be painful, and infected teeth and gums harboured infection in the mouth producing bacterial toxins believed to increase insanity. Rotten teeth were extracted.

Forced feeding

'Forcible' or 'artificial' feeding was viewed in some asylums as a remedy of last resort in patients who refused to eat. Patients would always be encouraged to take their food naturally. Forced feeding was used as a means to preserve life.

Loss of appetite was a common symptom in reaction to acute grief and in cases of melancholia. Persistent refusal to eat was also commonly seen in patients who had paranoid delusions that their food was poisoned. This idea occurred more frequently amongst private patients. If their delusion was that the food was poisoned, then the attendant could taste a small sample first to reassure the patient.

When forced feeding was deemed absolutely necessary, the first move would be an attempt to spoon-feed. A wooden spoon was placed in the mouth and gently rotated to a right angle to keep the mouth open, taking care not to break any teeth. Another spoon was used to place liquid or semi-solid food into the mouth. This was generally acceptable but gave the patient the opportunity to spit the food out.

If this method failed, more invasive methods of feeding would be used, sometimes necessitating the use of a stomach pump. The patients would be given liquid nutrients directly into their stomachs via a rubber tube that was over 2ft long and passed through either their mouth or nose; the medical superintendent carried out the delicate procedure, which could not be left to staff or attendants. Liquidised food was passed through this tube via a funnel (relying on gravity), a syringe, or a mechanical pump. The advantage of the nasal tube was that it could be used in patients who firmly clenched their teeth shut, and it would not damage any teeth. The patients did not usually agree to this form of 'therapy' and often had to be physically restrained during the process – this required the patient to be wrapped tightly in a sheet to restrict movements of their arms and legs, and being held down by four attendants – one at either side, one to control the head, which would be firmly held within a towel placed between that attendant's knees, and another to control the feeding.

Foodstuffs used for forced feeding included: beef tea, raw eggs, ground meat, custards, milk, pearl barley, strong ale, diluted brandy and

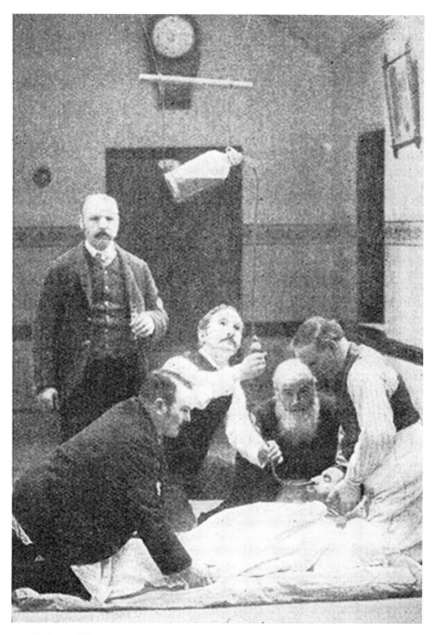

Dr William Whittington Herbert force-feeding a patient at Denbigh Asylum. British Medical Journal, 1894.

sherry. Private patients were occasionally fed with champagne, turtle soup, concentrated chicken and oyster broths.

Often when an obstinate or hysterical patient was shown the feeding apparatus and had the process of forced feeding explained to them, they would give in and eat.

Case study: Alice Ashton

Alice Ann Ashton, a 19-year-old from Stockport, was rambling incoherently when she was admitted in July 1892 with epileptic mania. She was extremely obstinate and self-willed and would not reply to any questions. Alice was noted to be 'untidy in her dress and […] constantly spitting at people without warning. She absolutely refuse[d] to take any food whatever and ha[d] to be fed with the tube.' Alice required frequent seclusion for violent, quarrelsome and unmanageable behaviour, but after three days of nasogastric tube feeding, she opted to take her food naturally again. Alice was regularly secluded during her stay in the asylum for violent, uncontrollable outbursts. She died without improvement on 13 January 1901 from phthisis pulmonalis (tuberculosis).

Case study: Helena Burgess

Helena Burgess was a 50-year-old widowed shopkeeper from Angleton when she was admitted to an asylum on 12 September 1894 suffering from acute mania. Her refusal to eat led to her being forcibly fed by a tube until eventually she could be fed by the asylum attendants from a spoon. Mental relapses within the asylum inevitably resulted in her refusal to eat and she was tube fed on several more occasions. She died on 31 May 1899 from chronic Brights disease (kidney failure).

Mesmerism

Mesmerism was similar to hypnotism and was introduced by the German physician Franz Anton Mesmer (1734–1815) who believed that magnetic forces within a person could be harnessed and channelled. The therapist looked fixedly into the patient's eyes and moved his hands near their body, or placed them on their abdomen. As late as 1881, restraint was still being used in Exeter to tie 'violent' patients with cords onto a 'revolving bed' so that mesmerism could be administered, albeit as part of a series of experiments.

TREATMENTS

Electricity

The application of electric currents as a medical therapy was experimented with in the late nineteenth century. Two types of electric current were identified: contact-electricity (direct current or DC) was discovered in 1789 by Luigi Galvani (1737–98) electromagnetic induction (alternating current or AC) was discovered in 1832 by Michael Faraday (1791–1867). Constant galvanic currents could be provided by galvanic batteries, and alternating faradic currents were produced by magnetism or induction. Repeated applications of 'galvanism' were found to be beneficial in some functional (as opposed to organic) mental disorders. Electricity was seen as a powerful, stimulating adjuvant to other treatments. This use of electricity was very different from electroconvulsive therapy (ECT), which was not introduced until the twentieth century.

Case Study: Margaret Young

Margaret Young, a 44-year-old unmarried fieldworker, was suffering from chronic mania. Her asylum notes record that, on 1 July 1891:

> *magneto-electric current was applied to her, the electrodes being, one in a porcelain foot bath, the other applied over various parts of her scalp and spine. The effect of it is to make her decidedly more lively and biddable and greatly to increase her appetite for food, which she eats ravenously after the application.*

Alcohol

Alcohol was used in some asylums to stimulate appetite and promote sleep. Alcoholic spirits, usually brandy or whisky, were used medicinally to soothe patients when they were dying.

Case studies: alcohol

When the demented 62-year-old Mary Archer succumbed to erysipelas in Parkside Asylum in 1872 and was on her deathbed, she was prescribed 'one teaspoon of whisky every three hours'.

Mary Rutherford, aged 79, was admitted to the Roxburgh Asylum in December 1898 suffering from senile dementia; 'excited, voluble and very communicative'. On 9 January 1899 her breathing became slow and shallow. Her case notes record – 'warmth was applied to her extremities and Brandy administered. She died at 12.25 am.

Moral therapy

Reforms in the treatment of the insane at the end of the eighteenth and beginning of the nineteenth centuries led to what became known as 'moral therapy' or 'moral treatment'. Patients were removed from the environment where their disease had developed and placed in a safe and humane environment where they could receive proper care and attention. Moral therapy was based on restraint by kindness and understanding, rather than restraint by manacles or other physical restraints – they were managed by a system of designed techniques including rewards and punishments, reason, and emotion. It embodied the principles and importance of a good doctor-patient relationship. It was based on an intensive, individual psycho-therapeutic approach, akin to modern cognitive behavioural therapy. The controlled environment encouraged patients to collaborate in their own treatment and recovery. The asylums were run with an orderly routine, staffed by competent, trained and well-supervised attendants. It could be seen as a form of behavioural therapy but drugs were also used. In the early nineteenth century, moral therapy was viewed with scepticism as many people, including many of the asylum staff, believed that the insane were no better than animals and should be treated as if they were dangerous and threatening and therefore be restrained.

Moral, humane therapy is said to have been developed at the Quaker foundation of the York Retreat, which opened in 1796, but there is evidence that it was already well established at the Ticehurst private asylum in Sussex by 1792. Robert Gardiner Hill (1811–78), house surgeon at the Lincoln Lunatic Asylum, introduced moral therapy there, writing in 1838: 'Restraint is never necessary, never justified, and always injurious, and its application consequently unjustified.'

Gardiner Hill removed the patients' leg irons and straight-jackets. Following the successful use of moral therapy at the large metropolitan Middlesex County Asylum at Hanwell in the 1840s and its promotion by Dr John Conolly, it widely became accepted as the best way forward for the management of the insane.

The District Asylums in Scotland and the new county asylums in England and Wales developed into self-sufficient communities with their own farms, gardens, workshops, and other industries. Rather than being established within cities, these new district asylums were established in the rural countryside, on the outskirts of towns where there was a surplus of land to provide full agricultural employment for the male patients.

Inmates were encouraged to feel that they were useful members of the asylum community, as this would contribute to repairing their self-esteem and regaining their lost reasoning. For males, agricultural labour, when combined with an adequate diet, was thought to improve recovery. The females worked in the laundries, or in the sewing or knitting rooms making and repairing clothes. They helped in the kitchens, and by cleaning wards. The men acted as farm labourers or market gardeners, or were employed as craftsmen in workshops. Archives from the Roxburgh District Asylum record men employed as shoemakers, tailors, blacksmiths, carpenters, joiners, masons and upholsterers. The collective action of people working together must have fulfilled a social function that would also have been therapeutic. Some cynical commentators have argued that the work carried out by inmates was mainly for the economic benefit of the institutions, and was used as a method of controlling them. Recreation, exercise and amusement in the asylums was also encouraged, including country walks, weekly dances, concerts, theatrical performances, lectures, board games, various sporting activities, regular excursions and occasional picnics. The asylums held extensive libraries for the use of their inmates and newspapers were also provided.

Religious services were held every Sunday with the two sexes sitting apart yet in view of each other, except at Perth where a partition divided the room into two compartments, with half of the pulpit in each.

However, as the nineteenth century progressed it became increasingly apparent that moral therapy was overly optimistic and completely doomed to failure – most patients were not cured and did not return from the asylum as valuable members contributing to their communities. There was a growing, pessimistic realisation that lunacy and learning disabilities were possibly inherited and often incurable.

The Lunacy Commission reported in 1901:

Now the asylums are congested with aged, infirm and broken down persons and vacancies for acute cases are difficult to secure ... resources are largely monopolized by the class to which we have referred, many of whom do not need its costly appliances, and were not benefited by its hospital appliances, and which are not benefited by its hospital equipment, and they crowd out those who are urgently in need of both.

Drug therapy

Sedatives and hypnotics
Patients were frequently sedated. Sedation was used to reduce tension and anxiety and to induce calm, and also to give some respite to their attendants. Usually a combination of the sedative agents listed below was used as a cocktail. Sleep was viewed as essential for resting and repairing the body and hypnotics were used to induce sleep.

Bromides
Bromide salts, particularly potassium bromide, were often used as sedatives in the nineteenth and early twentieth centuries. The sedative virtues of the bromides were extolled by the obstetrician Sir Charles Locock (1799–1875) in his contribution to the 1857 meeting of the Royal Medical and Chirurgical Society in London. Locock described: the anticonvulsant effects of the bromides and talked about how he had used them to stop epileptic seizures in 'hysterical' women. Potassium bromide was undoubtedly the first effective medicine used to treat epilepsy, initially used for that purpose in the 1850s. Locock also considered that the bromides repressed sexual excitement – leading him to believe that this was why potassium bromide was successful in treating seizures. Sodium bromide was also effective for treating epilepsy and insomnia.

Chloral Hydrate
Chloral was used as a sedative and hypnotic. Introduced in 1869, it is a derivative of ethyl alcohol and was the first synthetically produced drug to treat insomnia. It did not produce the gastro-intestinal side effects of opiates but did slow the heart beat and lower the rate of respiration. In the 1890s, chloral hydrate was the most effective treatment for prolonged convulsion (*status epilepticus*).

Chloroform
Chloroform became popular from the 1850s onwards after it had been used by the Scottish obstetrician, Sir James Young Simpson (1811–70), for pain relief during the births of Queen Victoria's last two children. Chloroform vapours were used as inhaled anaesthetics to relieve pain and also to induce unconsciousness. It was sometimes used to sedate unruly

patients whilst bringing them from their homes into the asylum, and occasionally used prior to forced feeding. Ether had a similar action.

Hyoscine
A drug used as a treatment for motion sickness; it also reduces nausea, and sweating but causes a dry mouth. It was used in the treatment of acute mania.

Opiates
Opium, morphine and codeine were widely used as painkillers, pick-me-ups and nerve-calmers. However, these narcotic drugs could stimulate over-excitement and had the side effect of causing constipation. They were also addictive.

Paraldehyde
Paraldehyde was introduced into the United Kingdom in the early 1880s. It is an anticonvulsant, hypnotic and sedative. It was mainly used as a hypnotic and was found to be particularly useful for inducing sleep in patients suffering from delirium tremens (DTs) in alcohol withdrawal; it had an unpleasant taste and gave a disagreeable odour to the patient's breath. Paraldehyde could not be used in patients suffering from phthisis as it caused coughing and vomiting in these cases.

Sulphonal
The hypnotic sulphonal was introduced in the 1890s as an alternative to chloral with fewer side effects. It was not quite as effective as chloral hydrate in inducing sleep, taking longer to act and causing drowsiness the day after administration, but was considered a much safer drug.

Tincture of Cannabis
Tincture of cannabis was made by soaking the dried flowers of the Indian hemp plant (marijuana) in alcohol. It was used to treat melancholia by converting the depression into exaltation, usually inducing pleasant excitement. However, it could also cause hallucinations.

Chapter 20

Biographies

Ashley-Cooper, Anthony, 7th Earl of Shaftesbury. Born 28 April 1801, Grosvenor Square, London. Died 1 October 1885, Folkestone, Kent. English politician, philanthropist and social reformer. Educated Harrow School and Christ Church, Oxford. Styled Lord Ashley 1811–51, then Lord Shaftesbury 1851–85. Tory Member of Parliament for Woodstock, Oxfordshire from 1826, and for Dorchester from 1830. Member of the Select Committees on Pauper Lunacy in Middlesex and on Lunatic Asylums. Instrumental in setting out the *County Lunatics Asylum Act* of 1828 and the 1828 *Madhouses Act*. Commissioner in Lunacy; Chairman Metropolitan Commission on Lunacy, 1833; Permanent Chairman of the Lunacy Commission, 1845–85. Sponsored the two *Lunacy Acts* of 1845.

Browne, William Alexander Francis. Born 24 June 1805, Stirling, Stirlingshire. Died 2 March 1885, Crindan, Dumfries, Dumfriesshire. Asylum reformer. After graduation in medicine at the University of Edinburgh in 1826 he went to France to study mental illness under J.E.D. Esquirol (1772–1840) at La Salpêtrière. Fellow of the Royal Medical Society, 1825. Medical superintendent, Royal Lunatic Asylum, Montrose, 1834–38, where he introduced moral treatment. Doctor of Medicine, Heidelberg, 1839. Medical superintendent, Crichton Royal Institute, Dumfries, 1838–57. Commissioner for Lunacy for Scotland, 1857–70. President, Medico-Psychological Association, 1865–66. Author: *What asylums were, are, and ought to be* (1837). This text played a significant part in the reform of the asylum system and the treatment of lunatics in Great Britain and Ireland in the nineteenth century.

Bucknill, John Charles. Born 25 December 1817, Market Bosworth, Leicestershire. Died 19 July 1897, Bournemouth, Dorset. Psychiatrist and mental health reformer. Graduated bachelor of medicine, University

College, London, 1840. Medical superintendent, Devon County Asylum, Exminster, 1844–62. Lord Chancellor's Visitor in Lunacy, 1862–76. Fellow of the Royal Society, 1866. Founder *Asylum Journal*, 1853, which became the *Journal of Mental Science* (Editor, 1853–62). Co-author, with Daniel Hack Tuke: *A Manual of Psychological Medicine* (1858). Author: *Notes on Asylums for the Insane in America* (1875). Knighted 1894.

Clouston, Thomas Smith. Born 22 April 1840, Birsay, Orkney. Died 19 April 1915, Edinburgh, Midlothian. Graduated Doctor of Medicine, University of Edinburgh, 1861. Medical superintendent, Cumberland and Westmoreland Asylum, Carlisle, 1863–73. Medical superintendent, Royal Edinburgh Asylum, 1873–1908. Lecturer on mental diseases, University of Edinburgh, 1879–1908. President, Medico-Psychological Association, 1888. President, Royal College of Physicians of Edinburgh, 1902–04. Author: *Clinical Lectures on Mental Diseases* (1883); *The Neurosis of Development* (1891); *Unsoundness of Mind* (1911). Knighted 1911.

Conolly, John. Born 27 May 1794, Market Rasen, Lincolnshire. Died 5 March 1866, Hanwell, Middlesex. Graduated Doctor of Medicine, University of Edinburgh, 1821. Professor of the nature and treatment of diseases, University of London, 1828–30. Resident physician, Middlesex County Asylum, Hanwell, 1839–44. Visiting physician at Hanwell, 1844–52. At Hanwell, Conolly introduced the principal and practice of non-restraint in the treatment of the insane. Author: *An Inquiry into the Indications of Insanity* (1830); *Construction and Government of Lunatic Asylums* (1847); *The Treatment of the Insane without Mechanical Restraints* (1856).

Crichton-Browne, James. Son of Dr William A.F. Browne (see above). Born 29 November 1840, Edinburgh, Midlothian. Died 31 January 1938, Dumfries, Dumfriesshire. Medical superintendent, Newcastle-upon-Tyne Asylum, 1865–66. Graduated Bachelor of Medicine, University of Edinburgh, 1862. Medical director, West Riding Lunatic Asylum, Wakefield, Yorkshire, 1866–75 from where he taught psychiatry to students from the Leeds School of Medicine. Lord Chancellor's Visitor in Lunacy, 1875–1922. President, Medico-Psychological Association, 1878. Elected Fellow of the Royal Society, 1883. Knighted, 1886. He was widely honoured on his death in 1938 as 'the last of the great Victorians'.

Dix, Dorothea Lynde. Born 4 April 1802, Hampden, Maine, USA. Died 17 July 1887, Cambridge, Massachusetts, USA. An American educator, social reformer and activist who campaigned for asylum reform throughout America. She visited Scotland and Jersey in 1855 and lobbied the Westminster government to impose the English model of publically funded, centrally supervised, pauper asylums on the Scots. She was successful in lobbying Queen Victoria and Parliament for improvements to the asylum system in Jersey.

Down, John Langdon. Born 18 November 1828, Torpoint, Cornwall. Died 7 October 1896, Normansfield, Middlesex. Medical superintendent at the Earlswood Asylum for Idiots at Redhill, Surrey, 1858–68. Established Normansfield, 1868 – a private institute for children with learning disabilities at Hampton Wick. Described Down's syndrome, 1866. Author: *Observations on an ethnic classification of idiots* (1866); *On some Mental Affections of Childhood and Youth* (1887).

Duncan, Andrew. Born Pinkerton, near St Andrews, Fife, 17 October 1744. Died 5 July 1828, Edinburgh, Midlothian. President, Royal Medical Society, 1767 and 1769–74. Doctor of Medicine, University of St Andrews, 1769. President, Royal College of Physicians of Edinburgh, 1790. Proposed the erection of a public lunatic asylum for Edinburgh in 1792, which was finally built at Morningside in 1807 and became the Royal Edinburgh Asylum. He was awarded the Freedom of Edinburgh in 1808. Author: *Elements of Therapeutics* (1770).

Ellis, William Charles. Born 10 March 1780, Alford, Lincolnshire. Died 24 October 1839, Southall Park. Medical superintendent at the West Riding Pauper Lunatic Asylum at Wakefield, 1817–31, and the first medical superintendent at the Middlesex County Asylum at Hanwell, 1831–38. Ellis and his wife Mildred were devout Methodists who ran the asylums they had charge of with humane and moral treatment. He became famous for his pioneering work and was awarded a knighthood. Author: *A Treatise on the Nature, Symptoms, Causes and Treatment of Insanity, with Practical Observations on Lunatic Asylums: And a Description of the Lunatic Asylum at Hanwell* (1838).

BIOGRAPHIES

Gardiner Hill, Robert. Born 26 February 1811, Louth, Lincolnshire. Died 30 May 1878, Earl's Court House, London. Member of the College of Surgeons, 1834. Appointed resident house surgeon to the Lincoln Lunatic Asylum, 1835–40, where he introduced a method of 'non-restraint' by removing patients' handcuffs, leg irons and straight-jackets. This had a profound influence on John Conolly, who employed the same method on his patients at Hanwell. Author: *A Concise History of the Entire Abolition of Mechanical Restraint in the Treatment of the Insane* (1857).

Haslam, John. Born 1764, London. Died 20 July 1844, London. Resident Apothecary at Bethlehem Hospital who was dismissed from his post following the 1815 Select Committee Enquiry into the State of Asylums in England and Wales. He was created a Doctor of Medicine by the University of Aberdeen on 17 September 1816 and began a private practice in London. He published several papers, most notably: *Observations on Insanity, with Practical Remarks on the Disease and an Account of the Morbid Appearances on Dissection* (1798).

Holloway, Thomas. Born 22 September 1800, Devonport, Plymouth, Devon. Died 26 December 1883, Tittenhurst Park, Sunninghill, Berkshire. Philanthropist and inventor of patent medicines who financed Holloway Sanatorium in 1885 at Virginia Water, Surrey for 240 middle-class mentally ill patients, and Royal Holloway College – a college of the University of London in Egham, Surrey for the education of women in 1879. Both were gifts to the nation.

Hughlings Jackson, John. Born 4 April 1835, Green Hammerton, Yorkshire. Died 7 October 1911, Manchester Square, London. Fellow of the Royal College of Physicians and revered as the 'father of English neurology', Jackson was an eminent early neurologist who studied epilepsy. Doctor of Medicine, University of St Andrews, 1860. In 1862 he was appointed assistant physician, later (1869) full physician at the National Hospital for Paralysis and Epilepsy located in Queen Square, London. In 1878, together with Sir David Ferrier and Sir James Crichton-Browne (see above), Jackson was one of the founders of the important *Brain* journal, which was dedicated to the interaction between experimental and clinical neurology and is still published today. Localised focal epilepsy became known as Jacksonian epilepsy following his investigations into this type of convulsion.

Monro, James. Born 2 September 1680 in Wemyss, Fife, Scotland. Died 4 November 1752 at Sunninghill, Berkshire. Physician and specialist in insanity, James Monro was the first of four generations of Monros to hold the post of physician to Bridewell and Bethlehem Hospitals between 1728 and 1853. Graduated BA, Balliol College, Oxford, 1703; and, Bachelor of Medicine, 1709. Doctor of Medicine, 1722. Fellow of the Royal College of Physicians, 1729. Monro was appointed to Bethlehem Hospital on 9 October 1728. He made no contributions in writing on the subject of insanity and was much criticised for preventing visits by doctors and family members to patients within the hospital.

Monro, John. Born 16 November 1715 at Greenwich, Kent. Died 27 December 1791 in Hadley, near Barnet. Physician and eldest son of James Monro. Graduated Bachelor of Medicine, Oxford University, 1743. Fellow of the Royal College of Physicians, 1753. He succeeded his father as sole physician at Bethlehem Hospital in London in 1752. As well as his role as physician to Bethlehem, Monro also had interests in private madhouses in London, which provided him with a lucrative income.

Monro, Thomas. Born 1759, London. Died 14 May 1833 at Bushey. He was the youngest son of John Monro and became assistant physician to his father in 1787. Graduated Doctor of Medicine, Oriel College, Oxford, 1787. He succeeded his father as physician at Bethlehem Hospital in London in 1792. He attended King George III during his second bout of madness in 1811–12, in a joint consultation of independent 'specialists', with John Willis and Samuel Foart Simmons. He was also called on by counsel to give evidence concerning the state of mind of John Bellingham before the latter's trial for the assassination of the Prime Minister, Spencer Perceval, in 1812. Thomas Monro is perhaps best known for the damning evidence produced by the Select Committee Enquiry of 1815 into conditions at Bethlehem Hospital. Following this, Thomas stepped down in 1816 and his son Edward took over.

Quarrier, William. Born 16 September 1829 in Greenock, Renfrewshire. Died 16 October 1903 at Quarrier's Homes, Bridge of Weir,

Renfrewshire. Philanthropist and social reformer. Quarrier became fatherless at the age of 3 when his father died of cholera in Quebec. He started work in a pin factory in Glasgow when he was 6 and never forgot the hardship of his early life. He took a great interest in the plight of orphaned and destitute children in his home city of Glasgow and, with the help of friends, set up a couple of self-help groups – a Shoeblack Brigade which provided young boys with an income by polishing shoes, and a Parcel Brigade which carried parcels across Glasgow for tuppence a half mile or threepence a mile. His vision to assist all impoverished children helped him build homes for orphaned children in a specially created village colony at Bridge of Weir. Quarrier's village in Bridge of Weir grew and there were more than fifty houses, a school, church, dairy and poultry farms and workshops. Quarrier homes remain in existence today.

Skae, David. Born 5 July 1814, Edinburgh, Midlothian. Died 18 April 1873, Morningside, Edinburgh. Scottish alienist and physician. Fellow of the College of Surgeons of Edinburgh, 1836. Honorary Doctor of Medicine, University of St Andrews, 1842. Physician superintendent, Royal Edinburgh Asylum, 1846–73. Developed a classification of the various forms and a theory of the aetiologies of mental illness based on his so-called 'natural history of insanity'.

Tuke, Daniel Hack. Born 19 April 1827, St Lawrence Street, York. Died 5 March 1895, Marylebone, London. Youngest son of Samuel Tuke and Priscilla Hack. At the age of 20, he was appointed Secretary and House Steward to the York Retreat. Graduated Doctor of Medicine at Heidelberg in 1853. Physician and writer on psychological medicine. Visiting physician to the York Retreat, 1853. Editor of the *Journal of Mental Science* (1880). Co-author, with John Charles Bucknill: *A Manual of Psychological Medicine* (1858), which was regarded as the standard textbook on psychiatry for many years.

Tuke, Samuel. Born 31 July 1784, York, Yorkshire. Died 14 October 1857, York, Yorkshire. Quaker tea merchant, philanthropist and asylum reformer. Grandson of William Tuke and son of Henry Tuke who together co-founded The York Retreat. He wished to become a doctor but was directed into the family tea business. Acted as Treasurer of The Retreat,

1822–53. Author: at his father's request of *Description of the Retreat near York* (1813); *Practical Hints on the Construction and Economy of Pauper Lunatic Asylums* (1815); *Management of Hospitals for the Insane* (1841); and, *Review of the Early History of The Retreat* (1846).

Tuke, William. Born 24 March 1732, York, Yorkshire. Died 6 December 1822, York, Yorkshire. Quaker, tea-merchant and philanthropist. With the help of fellow Quakers, he was instrumental in founding The York Retreat, which opened in 1796. The Retreat advocated a more humane approach to the treatment of people with mental disorders that was to become known as 'moral therapy' following the brutal death of Hannah Mills, a Quaker woman in appalling conditions at the York Asylum.

White, Francis. Born 1787, Carrick-on-Suir, County Tipperary. Died August 1859, Dublin. Secretary to the General Board of Health of the City of Dublin during the cholera epidemic of 1832. Surgeon to Richmond Asylum, 1835. Medical superintendent, 1840. President, Royal College of Surgeons of Ireland, 1836. As Adviser to Sir Edward Sudger, the Lord Chancellor, White had a major input into the first Privy Council rules for the regulation of district asylums in Ireland. Inspector-General of Lunatic Asylums or Hospitals for the Insane, 1846–57. Retired due to serious injuries sustained in a railway accident at Dunkitt, County Waterford in November 1856.

Williams-Wynn, Charles Watkin. Born 9 October 1775, Llangedwyn, Denbighshire, Wales. Died 2 September 1850, Grafton Street, London. Second son of Sir Watkin Williams-Wynn, 4th Baronet of Wynnstay. Member of Parliament for Montgomeryshire, 1799–1850. Barrister, Lincoln's Inn, called to the bar 1798. Graduated Doctor of Common Laws, University of Oxford, 1810. A forward thinking British politician and Member of Parliament who promoted the *County Asylums Act* of 1808 leading it to be called 'Mr Wynn's Act'. Father of the House of Commons, 1847. He helped improve the county asylums acts in 1828 and 1842.

Glossary

Aetiology

The explanation or exposition of the origin or causation of a disease.

Alienist

The nineteenth century term for a medical practitioner who specialised in mental illness; an archaic term for a psychiatrist. Most asylum doctors in the nineteenth century would have been termed alienists.

Alzheimer's disease

An organic and progressive brain disease that causes impairment of memory and mental functioning leading to dementia. Over fifty per cent of people diagnosed with dementia in 2000 were and are wrongly labelled Alzheimer sufferers.

Asylum

An institution providing a place of refuge as a sanctuary for protection. Most asylums were established to provide for the mentally ill, but asylums were also established for orphans or for individuals needing a home because of a disability such as deafness or blindness.

Bedlam

Originally, 'bedlam' was a colloquial term used to refer to the Hospital of St Mary of Bethlehem in Bishopsgate, London, which accepted patients with mental illness and put them on show. In a more general sense, the noun bedlam referred to any institution caring for lunatics. The word 'bedlam' is now in general usage to describe madness.

Bridewell

A house of correction or reform school for petty offenders. Named after the sixteenth

	century Holy Well establishment near St Bride's Well in London.
Compos Mentis	The legal term for soundness of mind, memory and understanding.
Congenital	A condition existing at (or prior to) birth.
Commissioners of Lunacy (England & Wales)	The Lunacy Commissioners had national authority over all asylums. The Commissions principal functions were to monitor the erection of public asylums, as required under the 1845 *County Asylums Act*, and to transfer all pauper lunatics from workhouses and outdoor relief to an asylum.
Criminal Lunatic	A person found not guilty of a crime by reason of mental incapacity or insanity.
Cretin	A person with physical deformities and learning disabilities caused by congenital hypothyroidism (thyroid deficiency). Cretins displayed stunted growth in both physical and mental aspects. Untreated congenital hypothyroidism could result in severe physical and mental impairment.
Delirium tremens (DTs)	A state of acute confusion caused by sudden withdrawal from heavy alcohol use. It often causes visual and auditory hallucinations and the physical signs of shaking, shivering and sweating.
Delusion	A false opinion or belief.
Dementia	'Dementia' covered a spectrum of disorders associated with an impairment of mental capacity and loss of memory reducing a

	sufferer's ability to perform activities of daily living.
Deranged	A popular term in the nineteenth century for someone insane.
Epidemiology	The study of the patterns, causes and effects of health and illnesses.
Epilepsy	A common yet serious neurological condition where there is a tendency to have seizures (convulsions, 'fits') arising in the brain.
Euphoria	A feeling of intense elevated mind and excitement; intense happiness.
Feeble-minded	A term used in the late nineteenth century to describe an individual with moderate learning difficulties considered to have a functioning ability above that of idiots and imbeciles.
General paralysis	Also known as general paresis or general paralysis of the insane (GPI). A progressive organic brain disorder caused by late-stage syphilis resulting in a variety of mental and physical symptoms such as dementia, psychosis, seizures and generalised muscle weakness.
Grand Jury	Irish legal body responsible for administration at county level.
Heritor	The proprietor of a heritable subject in Scotland. In Scots Law a heritor was liable for the payment of public burdens including poor rates amongst others.
Hallucination	Something perceived that is not actually present; a figment of the imagination.

Hallucinations can occur in all the senses – auditory, visual, smell, taste, or a sensation in or over the skin, guts or muscles.

House of industry | A charitable institution established after the Irish Poor Law to offer relief to the destitute in Ireland. Originally they took the form of workhouses where the poor were made to work in return for board and lodgings.

Idiot | An individual with profound congenital intellectual incapacity; generally considered to have an IQ less than twenty-five or mental age less than 3 years. They would have limited communication. Examples would include Down's syndrome (mongolism) or untreated cretinism (congenital hypothyroidism).

Imbecile | An individual who acquired moderate to severe intellectual impairment after birth; generally having an IQ of between twenty-six and fifty. Mental age less than 6 years.

Lactational insanity | Insanity induced by the onset of breast-feeding. A form of puerperal insanity.

Lunatic | A person who was born apparently normal but became mentally unstable in later years, often temporarily.

Mad-doctor | In the eighteenth and early nineteenth century this was the name given to a medically qualified physician or surgeon who cared for mentally unwell patients; it was an early title for a group of individuals who were later called 'alienists' and are today called psychiatrists.

Madhouse	Madhouses were the early private establishments that cared for mentally unwell people. The madhouses originated before private lunatic asylums and evolved into them as the medical discipline of psychiatry progressed.
Mania	A mental instability that may cause episodes of uncontrolled hyperactivity, fury, excitement, cheerfulness, euphoria or delirium.
Medical superintendent	The responsible physician or surgeon in charge of the patients and the administration of the asylum.
Melancholia	A mental instability leading to abnormal levels of depressed mood, anguish, feelings of dejection, mistrust or anxiety with loss of interest and pleasure in normal activities, loss of libido, disturbance of sleep or appetite, feelings of worthlessness and guilt, and thoughts of suicide or death.
Mental retardation	A degree of impairment of mental capacity caused by congenital deficiency or birth asphyxia. There is a spectrum of mental retardation.
Moral treatment	The delivery of therapy through compassion, understanding, sympathy and respect for the individual. Often described as 'restraint through kindness rather than restraint by chains'. Designed to induce patients to collaborate in their own recovery.
Pauper patient	A patient who, because of a lack of personal funds, had their maintenance costs paid for by their responsible parish or union out of poor rates.

Poorhouse	The Scottish equivalent of a workhouse. A house maintained by the parish for the poor living on public charity.
Procurator Fiscal	A law officer in Scotland acting as a public prosecutor with a remit including the investigation of all sudden and suspicious deaths. He could also order police cases directly to an asylum pending a sheriff's warrant.
Psychosis	A severe mental condition involving a 'loss of contact with reality' usually with hallucinations.
Puerperal	Of, relating to, or occurring within six weeks of childbirth.
Recovered	The patient was considered by the medical superintendent to be cured from their insanity as a result of treatment provided.
Retarded	*see* Mental retardation.
Relieved	The patient had relief from his symptoms, i.e. he had improved, but was not cured.
Sheriff	A Scottish law officer, equivalent to a judge in England or Wales.
Senile dementia	A common ageing process. Dementia or loss of memory (cognitive function) caused by old age.
Unrecovered	The patient who was neither recovered nor relieved. Unrecovered cases were often transferred to other institutions.
Workhouse	A public building where the very poor people of the parish received food and shelter in return for work.

Bibliography

Alty, Ann and Mason, Tom., *Seclusion and Mental Health, a break with the past*, (London: Chapman and Hall, 1994).

Andrews, Jonathan, Briggs, Ada, Porter, Roy, Tucker, Penny, and Waddington, Keir., *The History of Bethlem,* (London: Routledge, 1997).

Bartlett, Peter & Wright, David, eds., *Outside the walls of the asylum: The History of Care in the Community 1750-2000,* (London: The Athlone Press, 1999).

Broadhurst, David, *A History of Parkside Hospital Macclesfield 1871–1996: A Sense of Perspective*, (Leek: Churnet Valley Books 1997).

Cohen, Deborah, *Family Secrets: The Things We Tried to Hide,* (London: Penguin Books, 2014).

Cox, Catherine, *Negotiating Insanity in the Southeast of Ireland, 1820–1900,* (Manchester: Manchester University Press, 2012).

Davis, Gayle, *'The Cruel Madness of Love': Sex, Syphilis and Psychiatry in Scotland, 1880–1930,* (Amsterdam: Editions Rodopi B.V., 2008).

Davis, Mark, *West Riding Pauper Lunatic Asylum through time,* (Stroud: Amberley Publishing, 2013).

Eadie, Mervin and Bladin, Peter, *A Disease Once Sacred: A History of the Medical Understanding of Epilepsy*, (Eastleigh: John Libbey & Co Ltd, 2001).

Finnane, Mark, *Insanity and the Insane in Post-Famine Ireland,* (London: Croom Helm Ltd, 1981).

Higgs, Edward, *Making Sense of the Census Revisited*, (London: University of London, 2005).

Longmate, Norman, *The Workhouse,* (London: Pilmico, 2003).

243

Marland, Hiliary, *Dangerous Motherhood: Insanity and Childbirth in Victorian Britain,* (Basingstoke: Palgrave Macmillan, 2004).

Michael, Pamela, *Care and Treatment of the Mentally Ill in North Wales, 1800–2000*, (Cardiff: University of Wales Press, 2003).

Melling, Joseph and Forsythe, Bill, eds., *Insanity, Institutions and Society, 1800–1914: A social history of madness in comparative perspective,* (Abington: Routledge, 1999).

Porter, Roy, *Madness: A Brief History,* (Oxford: Oxford University Press, 2002).

Prior, Pauline M., *Madness and Murder: Gender, Crime and Mental Disorder in Nineteenth-Century Ireland,* (Dublin: Irish Academic Press, 2008).

Scull, Andrew, *Museums of Madness. The Social Organization of Insanity in Nineteenth-Century England,* (Harmondsworth: Penguin Books Ltd, 1982).

Scull, Andrew, *The Most Solitary of Afflictions: Madness and Society in Britain, 1700–1900,* (New Haven and London: Yale University Press, 1993).

Showalter, Elaine, *The Female Malady: Women, Madness and English Culture, 1830–1980,* (London: Virago Press, 1987).

Stirling, Jeannette, *Representing Epilepsy: Myth and Matter*, (Liverpool: Liverpool University Press, 2010).

Temkin, Owsei, *The Falling Sickness: A History of Epilepsy from the Greeks to the Beginnings of Modern Neurology*, (Baltimore and London: Johns Hopkins University Press, Revised edition, 1994).

Wheeler, Ian, *Fair Mile Hospital: A Victorian Asylum,* (Stroud: The History Press, 2015).

Wise, Sarah, *Inconvenient People: Lunacy, Liberty and the Mad-Doctors in Victorian England,* (London: Vintage Books, 2013).

Wright, David and Digby, Anne, eds., *From Idiocy to Mental Deficiency: Historical perspectives on people with learning disabilities,* (London and New York: Routledge, 1996).

Index

INDEX